Bringing Yoga to Life

The Everyday Practice of Enlightened Living

Donna Farhi

HarperOne
An Imprint of HarperCollinsPublishers

HarperOne

Permissions and credits appear on pages 249–250 and constitute as a continuation of this copyright page.

HarperCollins books may be purchased for educational, business, or sales promotional use. For information, please e-mail the Special Markets Department at SPsales@harpercollins.com.

HarperCollins Web site: http://www.harpercollins.com
HarperCollins®, 🔥®, and HarperOne™ are
trademarks of HarperCollins Publishers.

FIRST HARPERCOLLINS PAPERBACK EDITION
PUBLISHED IN 2004
Designed by Joseph Rutt

Library of Congress Cataloging-in-Publication Data
Farhi, Donna.
Bringing yoga to life : the everyday practice of enlightened living / Donna Farhi.
p. cm.
Includes bibliographical references.
ISBN: 978–0–06–075046–6
I. Yoga. I. Title.
RA781.F36 2003
613.7'046—dc21 2003050809

23 24 25 26 27 LBC 32 31 30 29 28

For Ray

Contents

Part 1

Coming Home

Chapter 1

We Begin Here

Monday night is the evening for beginners at the studio, and although it is only five-thirty the winter sky has begun to darken as students arrive, some tentatively, others in boisterous pairs who have egged each other on to come, and the silent furtive ones, not yet sure whether there is a special way to act when entering a Yoga school. Robin arrives a little late and searches nervously for the farthest corner, to hide behind the other attendees. "Why have you come?" I ask, and as we introduce ourselves Robin declares, with an edge of cynicism that I have grown to recognize as the thickening of skin over something far more tender, that she wants to lose a little weight, maybe learn to relax. "Seemed like a better option than ballroom dancing," she says smugly, raising a few eyebrows.

As the weeks go by, Robin begins to move forward in the room and to ask questions about the stiffness she feels in her back. "I don't know," she says offhandedly, "maybe it has something to do with my job. Some days I can hardly catch my breath." At the end of the first course Robin signs up for another, and months turn into years. A life is unveiled: an ambitious career, a marriage that didn't work out, a childhood much analyzed in therapy, and then an open question. How can this life become fresh again? How to peel away the veneer of self-defense and the sadness of disappointment? One summer Robin takes the leap and decides after much encouragement to attend a seven-day retreat. After a long and silent meditation one evening Robin comes to say good night, and we look into each other's eyes. Something ineffable is exchanged: a recognition that something important has been realized. For once Robin drops her guard, and without saying a word I sense a warmth and tenderness that belie her practiced bravado. This is not where Robin began, yet it is a place that has always been there awaiting her arrival.

Over two decades of teaching I have witnessed again and again the power that Yoga has to shift seemingly intransigent negative patterns and to awaken the body, mind, and heart to other possibilities. No matter who we are or how long we have been entrenched in self-defeating behaviors, through daily Yoga practice we can become present to our own fundamental goodness and the goodness of others. Rediscovering who we really are at our core opens the way to experiencing our most basic level of connection with others. This connectedness lies at the heart of the practice called Yoga. Living in a unitive state is not an esoteric concept, and it is not an elusive higher realm that only very clever people can aspire to. It is the opening of the heart so that we have the capacity to feel tenderness, joy, and sorrow without shutting down. It is the opening of the mind to an awareness that encompasses rather than excludes. It is the startling and immediate recognition of our basic sameness. It is the practice of observing clearly, listening acutely, and skillfully responding to the moment with all the compassion we can muster. And it is a homecoming with and in the body for it is only here that we can do all these things.

Counter to the plethora of seven-step solutions and quick-fix formulas offered by so many contemporary self-help guides, the ancient science of Yoga does not pretend to be simple, quick, or easy. It is a practice that takes into account the very messy and often complex phenomenon of what we call a human being and the equally challenging task of everyday living. What Yoga does promise, however, is that through sincere, skillful, and consistent practice, *anyone* can become peaceful, happy, and free. It does not matter who you are or who you take yourself to be. Neither does it matter what has happened to you in the past or where you find yourself in the present. Anyone who has the intention to break through self-limiting and self-immobilizing thoughts and behaviors can and will find freedom through this practice. Regardless if you are a beginner or an experienced practitioner, the moment you engage in Yoga practice you will discover that the practice is itself the reward. Peace of mind and freedom from fear are as imminent as your focus. This change of mind has immediate consequences. You start to feel a sense of ease with life, and you feel more able to adapt to change. You experience a new vitality and clarity that affect your relationships at home, at work, and in the world.

That we may have come to see ourselves as separate and shut off from others is the central dilemma that we methodically dismantle in our Yoga practice because it is from this false sense of separation that we create so much of our own suffering and contribute to the suffering around us. We begin by putting aside a little time each day so that we can deliberately slow down and in doing so find a more natural rhythm that supports our well-being. This more relaxed rhythm allows us to reflect rather than react, to soften rather than harden, and to see clearly how things are now rather than dwell on the past or worry about the future. We achieve this in Yoga practice by simple means. Through the practice of postures we release pent-up tensions that have accumulated in our body, and we further refine our physical senses so that we become sensitive, adaptive, and resilient. Simultaneously, we reacquaint ourselves with the cyclic nature of our breath and its relationship to the sensate wisdom of our body. We learn to inhale completely and open to new experience. We learn to exhale completely and let go of unnecessary tension and the past. And we learn to rest in the pauses in between this arising and dissolving cycle. Like a surfer out on the ocean swell, we start to align ourselves with the ebb and flow of life rather than fight with it. Gradually we begin to recognize that in between the ups and downs and the coming and going, there is a matrix of stillness that is the backdrop of all phenomena.

Through these embodied practices we also methodically and meticulously retrain the mind to work for us rather than against us. We learn to focus the mind on one thing at a time, and in doing so we can attend to our everyday tasks and responsibilities fully and effectively. Eventually, as we begin to wake up to what is actually happening in the here and now, we start to notice that there is something unchanging and reliable in between, beneath, and throughout our everyday experience, and when we can stay anchored in this awareness we don't get caught up and wrung out by things that previously bothered us. It is this silent yet vibrant backdrop running through all things that provides us with a tangible thread of connection between seemingly disparate elements. Finding this thread and dwelling in the connection are the hallmarks of the yogic experience.

Inside this more natural rhythm where there is time to pause, breathe, feel, and perceive clearly, we find that the most valuable thing we can ever possess is clearly within our sights: this life itself. We may notice that while life has been living itself through us, we have been absent from the experience. Where did we go, and how can we come home to the larger life that is possible for us?

However we may have squandered our inheritance as a human being, we will find the practices forgiving and compassionate. Our first forays into practice may reward us with an immediate experience of peace, serenity, and homecoming. We may feel awe at all the exhilarating new sensations and insights that accompany our practice. As in every reunion, however, there is also the recognition of what may have been forgotten, what has happened during the time of exile, and what now needs to be reclaimed. Like a child who has waited too long for an overdue parent, we may feel anger or grief that we have neglected ourselves for so long. "I can't believe I let myself get like this," students say, shocked to discover at the relatively young age of twenty or thirty that their bodies feel like deck chairs left out over a long winter. It may seem as if the body is an undifferentiated block of solid substance and we the owners have a blurry recognition of it at that. We may find that the heart has become hardened and bitter and that our minds may be perpetually scattered.

There is nothing particularly romantic or pleasant about these first encounters with a long-neglected self. We may have a vague idea that some reunion is taking place, but with whom? And how? Forget the tantalizing promise of chakras whirling in precise synchronization or the rise of kundalini up the spine. We're talking screaming hamstrings, spinal columns that sag in all the wrong places, arms that tire after a few seconds of being raised, and a mind that can't get past three on a count of ten without losing track. We're still trying to determine where our hip joint is and how to move it when the teacher has long since progressed to finer points. We're told to pay attention to our inhalation and exhalation, and it soon becomes apparent we're not sure which is which. Whether we are just beginning or have practiced for years, a hefty dose of humor and some well-placed self-acceptance will go a long way toward softening the blow of insight. What we are experiencing is absolutely predictable and normal. We are starting to wake up, and as the old plumber's adage goes, the first water coming out the pipe is not sparkling clear.

If we have been in exile from our self for a long time, when we begin this waking-up process we may encounter a poignant nostalgia for what we missed all those years. Our teacher demonstrates a posture with the agility of a cat, and we recall the time when we were limber and felt a natural connection to life. What did we give up in the process of becoming a responsible adult? And to what degree has our accumulated experience overshadowed wonder and delight with the stultifying instrument of cynicism? As we release long-held tensions, we may also dredge up old memories and negative patterns of thought and behavior that have plagued our lives. Even if we are well established in our spiritual practice, we may encounter new and sometimes frightening recognitions of our own mistruths, and with time these self-perpetuated delusions become more difficult to defend. Yet, if we could not have imagined the Pandora's box that lay waiting when we signed up for our first Yoga class, neither could we imagine the ease and the lightness of being we feel after only a few hours of this remarkable practice.

We may realize that we have spent the better part of our lives investing most of our time and energy in trying to secure this very feeling of lightness and wellness. We may have looked to others or to possessions to validate and uphold our sense of self. When we relinquish these misdirected efforts, we can turn our energies instead toward finding enduring peace and happiness. This is heartening news because it means that each of us has all the time and energy we need to embark on this path of peacefulness. It is through the technology of Yoga that we learn how to contain and liberate our energy and ultimately direct it toward a more positive way of being.

And what is this more positive way of being? When we are in full command of our physical, mental, and emotional capacities and in complete possession of our self, we begin to live fearlessly and to open to new experiences, new possibilities, and new challenges. Then the energy that we may have previously squandered defending and fortifying a limited definition of self is mobilized to express our unique talents and abilities. These abilities can then be directed in such a way as to fulfill our personal destiny. We rise to the occasion, and the occasion is this life, right now, just as it is. Practicing Yoga does not eliminate life's challenges, and neither does it provide us with a convenient trap-door to escape from life's distractions. Instead, Yoga gives us the skills to meet life head-on with dignity and poise.

This book is written for people who have given up the fantasy that happiness is determined by luck and circumstance and have realized that a meaningful and fulfilling life is the result of skillful means and self-determination. A growing number of people find neither reassurance or confidence in the quick fix or the latest cathartic therapy. Having tested such reductionistic strategies and found them lacking, such people are ready to commit themselves to a path that offers incremental changes over the course of a lifetime yet *real* changes that are enduring. What Yoga does offer is a genuine and time-tested practice that has proven itself effective over centuries by people like you and me: ordinary people leading ordinary lives facing extraordinary challenges. Yoga offers us a pragmatic and realistic practice that helps us meet the most difficult situations with courage and equanimity. Yoga does not remove us from the reality or responsibilities of everyday life but rather places our feet firmly and resolutely in the practical ground of experience. We don't transcend our lives; we return to the life we left behind in the hopes of something better.

And this ill-defined yearning for something better is what often moves us further and further away from our true self. In part 1 I beckon you to look deeply at this yearning and to define the source of this longing. Contained within that longing you will find your true motivation for practicing Yoga. In finding this true motivation, you open the way toward clarifying your intention so that you can use the life you have been given joyfully and for the benefit of others. More important, you will be able to recognize if you are using your Yoga practice to look at your life or to escape from it.

In part 2 we explore the means of attaining clear insight using as our guide the eight-limb path of Ashtanga Yoga proposed by Patanjali. Patanjali was a third-century B.C.E. Indian mystic and philosopher to whom is attributed one of the great Indian texts: the Yoga-Sutra, a collection of 196 aphorisms outlining eight limbs in the practice of Yoga. These limbs show us how the practices can be made relevant to daily life. The first two limbs, the *yamas* and *niyamas*, or ethical precepts for right living, act as the hub from which all the other limbs grow. In particular, we shall see that the *asana* practice, or the practice of physical poses, which has become popular in recent years, can effect deep change only when practiced within this larger context. We shall see that Yoga has less to do with standing on our head than standing on our own two feet and that the physical practices of Yoga remain mechanical gymnastics until transmuted by our intention to clarify the mind and open the heart. The *yama* and *niyama* prerequisite principles for living thus lay a foundation that will serve every aspect of our life, on or off the mat or meditation cushion.

As well as exploring the attitudes and practices that support the foundations of authentic Yoga practice, in part 3 we take a look at the many obstacles and distractions that will undoubtedly rear their heads along the way. These temporary roadblocks are predictable and often necessary components of any serious spiritual endeavor. Obstacles offer us an opportunity to rub up against what makes us uncomfortable instead of using our practice as a means of evasion. Grappling with these challenges is a sign, not that we are failing in our spiritual practice, but that we are deepening our humanity and thereby making for ourselves an anchor that keeps us tethered to the here and now.

Finally, we turn outward the inner focus that has been so necessary to establishing a Yoga practice. We find that what began as a personal practice for our own benefit can change the very nature of our everyday life and the wider world in which we live. We discover that this self-reflective journey has not made our world smaller and more encapsulated but rather has dismantled our perception of separation. This new awareness allows us to see that no matter how different we may appear on the surface, we all share the same life. And it allows us to see that no matter how convinced we are of our own ideas, there is always another facet to consider. Such an undefended self can arise only out of the inner tempering process of daily practice. Such is the paradoxical virtue of practice. Through steeling and strengthening ourselves in the kiln of daily practice, we unleash our capacity to be vulnerable, tender, and open. The world is in desperate need of these qualities.

The teachings of Yoga describe many extraordinary states of consciousness and superhuman feats of control. Many erudite books have been written on these hypothetical states offering us glimpses of a world beyond. While attaining such hyperconscious states may be of some value, of far greater value are our attempts, however crude, to live with greater kindness and compassion in our everyday lives. Therefore, throughout this book I have focused on the relative nature of spiritual practice and in doing so have tried to look at the often confounding and painful ways in which we humans grapple with our very existence. The focus of this book is not on enlightenment as a means to transcendence but, as Venkatesananda, a translator of the Yoga-Sutra, declared, "enlightened everyday living." I welcome you into the sacred science, art, and practice of Yoga. May your practice bring you home.

Chapter 2

Motivation: What Brings Us to This Moment?

You are what your deep, driving desire is. As your desire is, so is your will. As your will is, so is your deed. As your deed is, so is your destiny.

BRIHADARANYAKA UPANISHAD 4.5
Translated by Eknath Easwaran

Almost all action is based at its root on a spiritual impulse. However unlikely this might appear, when we delve deeper we find that all people are motivated by the same desire to be happy. This deep-seated wish may remain on the level of an unconscious yearning, for we rarely acknowledge our real longing to feel truly alive and at peace. This secret wish may haunt our waking and dreaming hours, like a barely perceptible melody in the distance always just beyond the reach of our comprehension. While we may know that something is calling us, we may not be able to discern what this something is. And so we go about our lives, attending to the practical concerns of the everyday but always with an inner suspicion that a terribly crucial piece of the picture is missing.

The impulse to discover, to know, and to reclaim our divine birthright appears to be a trait shared by all of humanity since the beginning of time. That we have this unbidden impulse is a clear sign that we already know the treasure that lies within us. Yet as long as this desire remains a fleeting notion, relegated to the dark recesses of our unconscious life, our actions and their fruits are unlikely to quench this deep longing. In our unconscious quest for happiness, we will cast our net here and there, chasing the rainbows of the ephemeral, hoping to capture the promise of a better life and enjoy it not just momentarily but forever.

This quest, ironically impelled for all the right reasons, may lead us to search for lasting fulfillment in things that are wholly unsuited to the task: work or career, possessions, relationships, sexuality, or sadly, when we become desperate, through food, drugs, or alcohol. Or we may even use the material dimensions of our spiritual practice to bolster our confidence and assuage our ambitions. While some of our attempts to grasp happiness may be noble in themselves, we find that however successful we become in our career, however impressively we sculpt our physique, and whatever possessions we manage to procure, they can give us only temporary respite from our inner yearning. Our inability to attain immutable happiness may cause us to invest even more energy in pursuits whose dividends have already proven to fall short of our expectations. If only we worked harder, earned more money, lost that extra ten pounds, or found the perfect partner, maybe then we would feel good. Eventually and inevitably we have to conclude that these efforts have been unsuccessful. Like the young child on Christmas morning who, after madly tearing the wrapping off all the presents, stares moments later in bored confusion, we discover that these outer objects cannot animate us for long.

While the quest for happiness is not new, the cultural context in which it takes place is. Never before in history have humans been bombarded so relentlessly with advertising and media propaganda, which exploit their unconscious spiritual desires to serve the gods of consumerism and greed. We may sincerely want to live ethically and to find a right means of livelihood, but how do we do this in a climate of competitiveness in which we're told it's a dog-eat-dog world and that good guys finish last? How do we balance a conviction to live more simply with our five-year-old daughter's refusal to walk anywhere without Barbie-glitter high heels? We notice the telltale wrinkles and changes that come with aging and want desperately to accept and embrace ourselves just as we are, but the latest cosmetic surgery commercial campaign has left us with a subtle but undeniable feeling of insecurity about our inner worth. We may be inspired by people like Martin Luther King Jr. and feel elevated by spiritual texts, and yet when we listen to the news the heroes of our society seem to be sports champions, celebrities, and supermodels. Living in a world that has lost its inner compass is difficult, yet until we understand and take charge of our spiritual impulse we will remain vulnerable to these powers that would have us serve the pathology of the culture and in doing so become an indispensable part of the pathology itself.

Understanding how insidious these influences are will be imperative in preventing our spiritual practice from becoming an extension of our previous striving. If we fail to recognize when and how these influences creep in, we may find that we have simply traded one driven pursuit for another. We may have given up on having the perfect interior decor, but now we're obsessed with having the perfect Yoga posture. We've stopped battling it out in the boardroom, but now we mentally berate ourselves on the meditation cushion. If our spiritual practice is driven by a need to generate certainty and security, we will be sorely disappointed. All too often the same forces that have driven our material pursuits drive our spiritual ones. If our practice is driven by fear and the need to solidify our worldview, it will lead us down the familiar road to suffering.

If the life that we do have seems unrewarding and we're not ready to look deeply at the cause, our weekends and holiday times may provide an escape. Unfortunately, the life we leave behind is little altered by these excursions, a realization that becomes readily apparent the moment we unpack. Years ago I taught a regular Yoga class at a resort in Jamaica. Each week the resort would fill with single men and women (and probably some not-so-single participants), who at first would look slightly bewildered at their arrival in paradise. For a week they were to be treated to the suspended reality of constant entertainment, drinking, random and by all accounts frequent sexual liaisons, fantasy theme evenings, and various forms of fun and games designed to help them let go of their inhibitions. As one women enthused, "I'd never do this in my Chicago life!" The incited debauchery would come to an abrupt halt on the day of departure, when they realized they were going back to their "real" lives. The suspended animation over, they were now to return to the hell of that office in Chicago or the floundering marriage. The mood on these days was often funereal, contrasting starkly with that of the next batch of giddy arrivals. At first I had reservations about bringing the sacred art of Yoga into such a place. But after almost every class a few people would stay on and inquire how they might investigate this practice of Yoga once they returned home. Over time I came to observe that these were the same people who, after a few days of trying on hedonism for size, now found themselves sitting around the pool, perplexed and sad: having arrived in paradise, they still felt like hell.

Whether we are hooked on food, alcohol, drugs, sex, money, work, or fame, the impulse to lose ourselves in these things can be seen as a spiritual impulse. By *spiritual impulse*, I mean a desire to experience a lightness of being and transcendence that does not take us away from our everyday experience but exists within it. For surely, what we long for is not a world beyond this one (which for most of us would mean death), but to find some happiness within the perplexing conundrum of our everyday lives. We only have to read the works of people recovering from addictions to see that behind the trappings of disease lies a mystical yearning that is as authentic and urgent as that of any pilgrim. Somewhere underneath bingeing, starving, exercising, drinking, hallucinating, climaxing, and purchasing, we are desperately seeking a way home to our self. The longer we have been in exile from this true self, the more desperate the yearning and, often, the more desperate the means of attaining pleasure.

For many the motivation to begin, sustain, or deepen a spiritual practice comes in the midst of grappling with an inner ordering process. As we sift through our life experience we may notice that we consistently allow the urgent to override the important. We may realize that we have a deeply ingrained habit of giving the most time, energy, and commitment to things that ultimately are not very important and that leave us at the end of the day with little enduring satisfaction. We may feel as if we are working for a demanding unknown boss and that we have yet to receive a real paycheck. This path inevitably leads us to interior bankruptcy. Even when we've reached a profound degree of dissatisfaction, the cycle of reinvesting our best energy in outward pursuits is hard to break, and because of this it may take many years before we are willing to take ourselves and the idea of practice seriously.

As we wrestle with this inner ordering process, we start to define our values and set priorities accordingly. If we have been in the habit of making lists of things to do, we start to put maintaining peace of mind at the top of the list. If we have never dared to put ourselves on the list before, we may make our debut appearance. When we realize that the entity that we call our "self" is the clearinghouse for everything that will happen to us, we may wake up to the realization that attending to the inner hygiene of this self is the most important thing we could possibly do in this lifetime. Now we are ready to settle in for the long haul. We've decided we are ready to grow up, and we have reached the sobering realization that it is our life and that there is only one person who can do the work.

Like a bird who instinctively navigates thousands of miles each year to nest in the same branch in the same tree, something in us is always seeking this place of homecoming. And this something in us knows the exact location of this place of rest. The word *nostalgia* has its root in the phrase "pain for home," *noste* meaning family or home and *algia*, pain. The consequence of being in exile is a growing sense of nostalgia, a longing, a pain for home. It is this longing that impels us to find some way of living in which we will be welcomed back into the family of belonging.

Our search, however misguided it may appear on the surface, is not fruitless or unnecessary. Trying the thousands of strategies that *don't* work brings us closer to asking essential questions. We soon realize that we are not looking for some place, person, or thing, but some way of making the life that we have livable. When we come to this flash of insight, we realize that what we are seeking is an intimate relationship with the potent and paradoxically unknowable *animating force* that stands behind our own creation. We are in fact the living proof of this force. And what is more, in searching high and low, far and wide, we have become distanced from rather than intimate with the very thing we are seeking.

Yoga is a technology for removing the illusory veil that stands between us and the animating force of life. Time tested over centuries, it is an empirically grounded practice that meticulously prepares us to live in the full awareness and enjoyment of our divine birthright. Transcendence, lightness of being, freedom, and happiness are not things that we can attain; they are what we become and are. It is what we have always been and what we will always be. Right now, as your eyes flicker from word to word, your fingers moving exactly as you want them, your body is living evidence of this extraordinary life force: so complex and mysterious that the most advanced scientists in the world cannot replicate the workings of one of your eyes, let alone your ability to comprehend these words or form the thoughts that may follow. Through the practice of Yoga, we gradually shift our perspective until we can perceive the vast and vibrating aliveness of this matrix that stands behind and interpenetrates our very being.

This majestic view, however, is rarely what motivates our first forays into Yoga. On the contrary, it is because our view is blocked that we become curious. It is like being seated at a theatrical extravaganza knowing that something really special is happening onstage but we can't quite see it because we're sitting behind a woman wearing a tall hat. As we shift from side to side, we may get a glimpse now and then of the action onstage, but these momentary glimpses only further tantalize us. It is only when we are utterly fed up with the inadequate sight line that it may occur to us to change seats and in effect to *change our point of view*. This desire to see more clearly is what impels many of us to begin Yoga practice.

Or we're in pain and we're utterly sick of it. Perhaps we are en-countering the same problem over and over and we have a hunch that our state of mind has something to do with our predicament. As infuriating as it is, we humans seem to derive far greater moti-vation from pain than from joy, and it is this pain that brings us to practice. While many people are called to practice Yoga as the result of a major crisis such as a divorce, the failure of a business, or a serious injury, far more begin for seemingly banal reasons: to lose weight, to reduce stress, or simply to spend a rare quiet mo-ment away from the raucous chaos of a family household. None of these reasons is better or worse than another, but almost certainly, the greater the pain and the more serious our predicament, the more motivated we will be in our practice. If we are lucky, through the help of our teacher and the sheer efficacy of the teachings, we will discover that underneath the most casual interest lies a strong de-sire for healing and happiness.

I well remember the first day of a Yoga intensive I was leading in Auckland, New Zealand. The pace at the beginning of such a seminar is always deliberately slow to give people a chance to relax, open up their perception, and begin the process of inquiry. But one woman was clearly finding the pace infuriating. Although we were only thirty minutes into the first class, she appeared to be jumping out of her skin and began to interrupt, asking questions about when we were going to do more postures and exactly how vigorous was the rest of the intensive going to be. "Why," I asked, "are you con-cerned about this?" "Well," she stammered, "it's crucial that I burn a certain number of calories during Yoga practice each day." There are moments when a teacher sees lucidly into the core of a student. It is a radical thing to act at such a time, but not to do so is to miss a golden opportunity. "I wonder," I gently countered, taking her to one side, "if you could slow down and become quiet, whether you might begin to understand what is driving you to overeat?" At this, tears began to well in her eyes, and she shared that her entire Yoga practice up to this point had been compelled by a terrible fear of gaining weight. Would she be willing to look a little deeper to see the real impulse behind her practice, which was to heal?

When I began my own Yoga practice at the age of sixteen, I was but a year away from entering a phase of undiagnosed eating disorders, beginning with anorexia and progressing to an all-consuming conflictual relationship with food. This disorder would tyrannize my life well into my early twenties. On that fated day when Yoga was announced as a possible elective class at my high school, I did not know why I signed up, why I liked the class, or why I decided to practice every day on my own at home for an hour each afternoon. In retrospect, I can see that attending that Yoga class saved my life. My family had been hemorrhaging internally from a crisis that had shattered every member of the household, and now, years later, the family was coming apart at the seams. We were recent emigrants from the United States to the far-flung islands of New Zealand, and I found myself completely and utterly alone. Where might I go to feel safe and protected? What I discovered in the confines of my bedroom, behind closed doors each afternoon, was that while I was practicing Yoga I felt a rare calm, a palpable sense of control, and a goodness within my body that was deeply reassuring. Surely, had I not felt so abandoned I would not have been compelled to seek this solace. In the pure naïveté that is the gift of youth, I began to have a dialogue with a part of myself that seemed to be beyond the reach of my painful, everyday existence. While I was under the spell of my Yoga practice, I felt neither fear nor pain. Without knowing it consciously, I started to make daily contact with this inner entity that spoke a wordless language I could understand. I began to feel supported by this inner friend, whose company could be conjured miraculously through making my breath calm and regular and through slowly stretching and holding myself still. Most incredibly, despite my circumstances I began to feel an inexplicable sense of *belonging.* That this should occur without my having had any formal instruction in the philosophical underpinnings of Yoga is a testament to the efficacy of this practice. One does not have to understand

Yoga, any more than one must understand the universe, for it to work.

The practice of Yoga helps us connect with the part of ourselves that is always virgin and untouched: the place within us that can never be damaged. While pain may be the catalyst that brings us to Yoga practice, it is joy that renews our commitment. As our glimpses of calm and clarity become more frequent, and as our response to the challenges of life becomes more skillful, we wish to practice not simply to get ourselves out of a fix, but also to strengthen our connection with this base state of contentment. The joy that I refer to is not the climactic high we associate with excitement or stimulation, but a deep sense of awe and wonder that can suffuse the most ordinary things and the most ordinary moments. This joy arises out of our own intrinsic nature and does not depend on external circumstances. Thus one of the highest expressions of this state of being, *samadhi*, is translated most accurately not as *ecstasy*, which means "to stand outside the ordinary self," but *enstasy*, which means "to stand inside the Self."[1] Both translations are in a sense correct, as Georg Feuerstein points out in his book *The Yoga Tradition*, because it is not until we can extricate ourselves from the limited viewpoint of the ego-self that we can avail ourselves of the panoramic possibilities of the larger life that is possible for us.

A much-respected colleague shared with me how he had managed to put enough money aside to take a short sabbatical from the demands of work and family and commit himself completely to his Yoga practice. After a few months he was becoming strong and flexible in his body and was soon able to do the advanced postures that had previously eluded him. He began to master very difficult breathing techniques and was experiencing new depths in his meditation. But as his sabbatical neared its end he noticed a subtle yet nonetheless deep anxiety. Once he had to work again it was unlikely he would be able to sustain the advanced *asana* and *pranayama* practice he had attained during his sabbatical. He realized then that identifying in his practice with things that could be lost would always leave him susceptible to fear. Anything that could be taken away through sickness, aging, or life circumstances was not a very wise thing to stand on. It was then that he realized that the only security lay in using his Yoga practice to tether his awareness to the part of himself that was and is eternal. It is in this tethering of awareness to the unchanging core of our being that true security can be gained. We find that the only thing that is unchanging in this core of ourselves is the radiantly alive and constantly vibrating pulse of life. When we arrive in this place, we realize there is no center and no periphery, that we are in fact infinite and limitless.

As our practice deepens and we gain confidence and courage, we develop a growing appetite for this groundlessness. We start to yearn for a more liberated and open experience of ourselves, and we become more willing to let go of old handholds. We start to feel a resolute commitment to real freedom, and we become vigilant about things that offer the trappings of freedom but fall short of delivering the goods. It can take many challenging years of practice to reach this place because the vastness of this interior freedom grants us a life that is larger than anything we could have imagined. So this is what it means to be alive.

Yoga tells us that the soul is always inexorably drawn toward those things that will most reveal its true nature. When we are able to recognize our spiritual impulse for what it truly is and to harness that impulse with discriminating awareness, we will find our way home just as surely as a migrating bird finds its nest. As we shall see, this process of finding our way home is a gradual process, happening in increments over the course of a lifetime. This does not mean we progress toward this place of belonging, for we cannot progress toward something we already are. It is through practice, however, that we come to realize the very nearness of our own liberation.

Chapter 3

A Larger Life

All life is being lived.
Who is living it, then?
Is it the things themselves,
or something waiting inside them,
like an unplayed melody in a flute?

Rainer Maria Rilke, BOOK OF HOURS 2.12
Translated by Anita Barrows and Joanna Macy

The practice of Yoga avails us to the largest possible life. What is this larger life? It is characterized by fearlessness, awe, and enchantment. It is the feeling most of us had as young children, perhaps when we rolled down a grassy slope, leaped off a bridge, or nestled in the arms of a loving grandparent. It is the suspension of time that occurs when we are so immersed in an activity that we become it: we no longer paint, we are painting, dancing, reading, listening, lovemaking, or walking. It is an experience of belonging, of homecoming, and of reconciliation. It is an opening into what we cannot possibly know, explain, or define and giving ourselves to this mystery unreservedly even though we have no idea where it will lead us. It is an awakening to the intensity of life when we drop our guard, with the full knowledge that to love also opens us to sorrow and loss. It is a bearing in which we allow all the senses to become amplified to sensation: a light breeze caressing the skin, the coolness of water, the colors of neon lights at night. It is a state of being that is so compelling that even a fleeting instance of being this alive, no matter how many years ago, leaves us haunted.

The word *Yoga* is derived from the verbal root *yug,* which means "to bring together" or "to harness." *Yoga*, in essence, describes both a practice and a way of being in which we realize the inherent unity behind the multiplicity of life's expression. In Yoga there is a tacit understanding that while we may have a body, a personality, and a name, this little self that we have come to believe is the entirety of our being is only a small part of something larger. The sages called this larger life *brahman*, from the root *brih*, which means "to expand." What we expand into is a common ground of existence, which makes up the essence of everything—the force behind the wind, the movement of the tides, the sap moving through a tree, and the life force moving through all creatures. We expand to become what we already are. The yogis of old discovered that this macrocosmic larger Self, spelled with a capital to distinguish it from the confines of the individual personality, can be found by looking within the microcosmic little self. Variously known as the Absolute, the Center, God, the *atman*, or Self within the self: it is the irreducible essence of everything. And that everything is what you are. This is the premise of Yoga practice and the promise that there is a larger life to which we all belong.

The words we use are big and perhaps intimidating, yet this practice is for ordinary people leading ordinary lives who wish to take up the extraordinary challenge of awakening to their true nature. And the challenge exists, not outside our everyday life, but within it. When Erin first came to me for private Yoga lessons, she hoped that Yoga practice might help her cope with depression. A twenty-eight-year marriage in which she felt neither meaning or pleasure had left her feeling disconnected and numb. Now divorced and nearing her sixtieth year, Erin wanted something more from her remaining years. As Erin began to release her chronic tension, new life began to flow through her arms and legs. The pronounced hump in her upper back began to straighten so that she could see the world around her from a new perspective. One day she arrived for her lesson very excited. On the way to the studio she had noticed the wind brushing against her skin and found pleasure in this newfound sensation. She related with great joy that that very morning she had noticed herself delighting in the pleasure of a hot bath. "Nothing's changed, but everything has changed."

The teachings of Yoga speak to us of what it is possible to be as a human being. What greater achievement, what greater enlightenment, could we possible attain than to become a decent person? The person who stops to help us with a flat tire on a deserted road or the one who returns our wallet—this is the person who restores our faith in the goodness of human nature. Central to the spirit of the Yoga tradition is the uncompromising belief in this fundamental goodness: this goodness *is* our true nature. Because what is possible is within us, the yogic quest is not a vertical evolution toward something else or somewhere else but a spiraling involution in which the end marks the beginning. We do not move toward a new and improved version of ourselves; rather, we return to an undifferentiated, unbounded sense of self that is open and innocent. When we are guided by this undefended Self, this larger life becomes available to us and we become available to serve this larger life.

This would all be very simple except that humans tend to view the world as ending at the boundaries of the skin. Our sense of alienation arises when we believe there is a "me" in here, and the world is out there; "you" and "I," "us" and "them" form the templates of a divisive and defended existence. Through simple inquiries such as observing the breath, yogis found that the world out there is constantly entering and altering us every moment of the day, suffusing our cells with life, energizing our nerves, and emanating from the light behind our eyes. And what is more, on further investigation, they concluded that "we" are not only breathing this life, "it" is also breathing us.

There is a delightful parable about the sage Ribhu and his disciple Nidagha in which the teacher challenges his student's habitual perceptions and in doing so opens the window for the student to see the unity that lies behind the veil of appearances. It is the challenge we all face when we avert our gaze from a homeless person, when we omit a difficult relative from the Thanksgiving dinner roster, or when we secretly deride an obese person. Although Nidagha had been taught the truth of oneness, he lacked the conviction to follow the path of Yoga, so he settled instead on leading a life devoted to religious ceremony and ritual. In spite of Nidagha's lack of faith, his teacher, Ribhu, so loved him that he visited him occasionally to see whether he had outgrown his ritualism. To determine the true state of his disciple's awareness, Ribhu often visited in disguise.

On one such occasion Ribhu took on the guise of a poor peasant and visited the village while a royal procession was in full swing. Stepping beside Nidagha and leaning on his crude walking stick, he said, "Excuse me, kind sir. I'm told the king is in the procession. How wonderful. But where is the king?"

"There," said Nidagha, pointing his finger to the front of the procession, "the king is riding on top of the elephant."

"You say the king is on the elephant. But which is the king and which is the elephant?"

"What are you talking about! It's obvious. There, the man above is the king, and the animal below is the elephant. Why am I wasting my time with such an idiot!"

"Please forgive me. I am but an uneducated peasant. But you said 'above' and 'below.' What do you mean?"

Exasperated, Nidagha replied, "For heaven's sake, if you cannot understand the words, I shall have to show you. Bend forward, and you shall know soon enough!"

And so the disguised sage bent forward, and Nidagha climbed up onto his shoulders.

"See now, I am above and you are below! Do you get it now?"

"No, not quite," replied the peasant faintly. "You say you are the king and I am the elephant. I am below and you are above. King, elephant, above, and below I understand, but pray tell me what do you mean by *you* and *I*."

At this Nidagha realized his master's guise and fell at his master's feet, declaring that he now understood the disguise of form and how this prevents us from seeing the truth of our unitive state.[1]

How do we change our point of view so that we too can see and experience this unitive state? Like Nidagha, we change our point of view when we see that there is something that binds us to everything else and that there are, as my mentor often said, "no strangers in this world." We do this by focusing the mind on the unchanging and eternal part of ourselves, which is always present. At the same time, we learn to observe the constant parade of visitors on this backdrop without getting too friendly or hostile toward any of these temporary guests. We don't invite and we don't refuse, we don't suppress and we don't indulge, we just let these guests come and go. Through practice, we find that there is a neutral "witness" that perceives these passing phenomena but does not falsely take these manifestations to be an accurate representation of itself. Further, we learn that it is unwise to build the scaffolding of our identity upon these transient and impermanent aspects, for to do so is to base our security on fleeting apparitions. Instead, we found our identity on that which is eternal in us and therefore totally reliable. It is in cleaving to this larger identity that we find an entirely different kind of security.

Unfortunately, what we want is what we most fear: we yearn for a larger life, but we're not so sure we want the consequences. Thus our little self almost always perceives the recognition of this larger Self as a threat. There is a humorous list of Murphy's laws for Yoga teachers, which states that the student who just declared that taking the first Yoga class was the most amazing experience of his or her life will not show up for next week's class. We may find that in opening to this larger life it is bigger and more chaotic and more filled with intensity than we'd like, and the fear invoked by the possible spaciousness of such a life sends us running back to our old stomping grounds. Our very sense of separateness and feeling of being cut off may impel us to defend the life we know even if it is filled with misery. We may even feel that to open ourselves up to life is to risk self-annihilation. In truth, it is the purpose of Yoga to destroy this limited sense of self so that, like Erin, we can discover the joy not only of being alive, but of letting life be who we are.

The practice of Yoga is therefore characterized by a meticulous process of deconstruction in which we make it our top priority to find out who we really are. We try to remember who we were before we had a name, before likes and dislikes, before all the prejudices that come with a fixed identity. What is left when we remove all that is impermanent and transient? Yoga tells us that what is left is in essence the only thing worth having: a connection to the source of our very aliveness. The belief in this effulgent source of aliveness is not founded on blind faith but is based on centuries of empirical inquiries into the nature of consciousness, the ground of existence, and the inextricable relationship between the human and the divine. These experiments carried out by yogic seers and sages resulted in the discovery of a radiantly vibrant force that acts as a living matrix behind the seemingly fixed, solid, and separate objects that most of us take to be reality. Their discoveries, uncannily similar to those of modern physicists, revealed that things are not as they appear to be. Rather, things appear as we believe them to be and are fashioned largely by the unquestioned conditioning of our habitual minds. That we may see ourselves as cut off, separate, and disconnected is a function of this skewed perceptual process and not, as we mistake it to be, evidence that this is how things really are.

We may falsely assume that we have something to gain through holding on to our little life. Maybe we hate our job, but at least we feel secure with money in the bank. Maybe we've been in an unhappy relationship for years, but we'd rather stay put in our misery than face the terrifying prospect of being alone. Perhaps we've had a vision of what we *really* want to do, but we come up with a hundred excuses not to pursue our dream.

After years of working for an ungrateful boss, one of my students, Liam, felt a deep sense of fear whenever he thought about quitting. Liam was not only an exceptional worker who had been an asset to his company, he was also a remarkably kind and gracious man who had managed to balance his passion for his study of Yoga with the nitty-gritty reality of working as a construction foreman. I was convinced that Liam had all the skills he needed to find a better work situation, yet his fear of leaving his job reigned supreme. Finally, after years of overwork, Liam succumbed to cancer and while recovering from surgery had more time to reflect on his past and where he was going. It was during this period of time that he realized how precious his life was and that it was time to make a change.

Positioning ourselves to see and experience this more encompassing view does two things: it opens us to new possibilities and freedoms, and it also makes us more vulnerable and exposed. If you have ever stood in the best vantage point for seeing a panoramic, 360-degree view, you know that such a place is necessarily completely exposed to the elements. From here you will see everything, but also from here you will feel everything in the most vivid way: the wind, the sun, and the rain. While there is nothing wrong with living in a little house with no windows, it is unlikely that we would experience many new freedoms from this vantage point. But the metaphor stretches only so far, for in Yoga the panoramic view we are speaking of is the view *in*. This view into our selves, however, leads to a more global view outward. As we become bigger, so does the world in which we live.

Which viewpoint we adopt—seeing the world from the perspective of connection or separation—will determine all our interactions and how we interpret and give meaning to even the most ordinary moments. As long as we see the world from the viewpoint of separateness, we are doomed to a life of conflict and suffering. Or as the Brihadaranyaka Upanishad declares, "The universe confuses those who regard it as separate from the Self" (4.6).

The text explains:

> As long as there is separateness, one sees
> another as separate from oneself, hears
> another as separate from oneself, smells
> another as separate from oneself, speaks to
> another as separate from oneself, thinks of
> another as separate from oneself, knows

another as separate from oneself. But when
the Self is realized as the indivisible unity of
life, who can be seen by whom? (4.14)[2]

When we do not experience this unity as the truth of our being, all our thoughts and actions are propelled by a kind of involuntary ignorance. We just can't help ourselves! All of the volatile and destructive emotions—anger, jealousy, envy, greed, and hatred—are born of this involuntary ignorance in which we perceive an "other" and therefore a need to propagate and protect "our" self. When we pick up the newspaper or listen to the news, the violence and atrocities that affront us are born of this same involuntary ignorance. We say that we just can't understand these things, but such actions are readily comprehensible in light of our failure to see ourselves in intimate relationship to one another.

Patanjali, the author of the Yoga-Sutra, a treatise of 196 terse aphorisms that delineate the process of becoming whole, tells us that our true nature consists of ten qualities of goodness. When we are centered within our true nature, these qualities shine forth. The ten attributes, called the *yamas* and *niyamas*, are traditionally considered the ethical precepts that bind and underpin all the teachings of Yoga. Because of their centrality, the *yamas* and *niyamas* are listed as the first two of the eight traditional limbs of Ashtanga Yoga practice, and adherence to these observances precedes and supersedes all other practices. (Other limbs include *asana* practice, or the traditional poses of hatha Yoga; *pranayama*, or harmonious breathing; *dhyana*, or continuity of focus; and others.)[3] Given Patanjali's extremely logical and systematic presentation in the Yoga-Sutra, we can be sure that it is not a coincidence that these ethical precepts are given such a prominent position. They range from scrutinizing how we relate to others to intensely investigating the state of our inner life. Often seen as a list of dos and don'ts or interpreted as a series of commandments, the *yamas* and *niyamas* are actually *emphatic declarations of what we are when we are connected to our true nature.*[4]

The *yamas*, or "outer observances," and the *niyamas*, or "inner observances," are often referred to as the inner and outer "restraints." What we restrain, however, is not our inherent badness or wrongness but our inherent tendency to see ourselves as separate. It is this inherent tendency that causes us to act outside our true nature. When there is an "other," it becomes possible to do things such as stealing because we falsely believe that what happens to another is not our concern. But when there is a sense of unity, who is there to steal from but ourselves? When we feel connected to others, we find that we are naturally compassionate, *ahimsa*, and that the first *yama*, "not-harming," is not something we strive to be but something that we are. We see the essence of ourselves in the other and realize that the tenderness and forgiveness we so wish to have extended toward us is something that all humans long for. The second *yama*, truthfulness, or *satya*, is based on the understanding that honest communication and action form the bedrock of any healthy relationship, community, or government. When we are not true to our values and personal sense of integrity, we not only are untruthful to others, we lie to ourselves and undoubtedly cause great inner turmoil. When we feel confident of life's abundance, we are naturally generous and able to practice the third *yama*, *asteya*, or "not-stealing." This *yama* of generosity has been proven to me over and over again when staying with people in India and other third world countries. Having few material possessions compared to Westerners, they display great pleasure in sharing their meager resources. The fourth *yama*, *brahmacharya*, or "containment of sexual energy," tells us to use our sexual energy in a way that makes us feel more intimate not only with our partner, but with all of life. When we are connected to our divinity, how then can we use another for our own selfish desires or hurt another through our inability to contain our desires? Finally, the fifth *yama*, *aparigraha*, or "not-grasping," tells us that letting go of all our embroidered images and identities is a sure way to realize the open nature of the mind. The veritable retinue of foot soldiers we procure in the way of objects, roles, and images, whether they be the right clothes or the right address, simply act to obscure our true nature. We're told that even if these identities and roles are part of our everyday life, they need not encumber us, and they can never be a true reflection of our absolute nature.

The "inner observances," or *niyamas*, act as a code for living soulfully. They tell us that when we are true to the highest expression of ourselves as humans, we live with *shaucha*, "purity," not because we're a Goody Two-shoes, but because it is the surest way to live life at a higher resolution with more clarity and happiness. If we fill our bodies with toxic substances and our minds and emotions with negative thoughts, we really can't enjoy this life we have. Purifying ourselves allows us to more easily practice the second *niyama*, contentment, or *santosha*. We find that all that we need lies within the content of the moment, even if that moment is difficult. This contentment arises out of a realization that no matter how sticky and difficult life can be at times, when we stand in our center our inner self remains essentially the same. This realization has enabled people living in prisons and in atrocious circumstances to maintain their dignity and poise and thus rise above their situations. To remain centered in this awareness takes discipline and enthusiasm, and thus *tapas*, or the "fire" or "heat" of spiritual practice, the third *niyama*, becomes a way of constantly clearing our slate of the daily residue that can color our perceptions. All of these practices require and encourage "self-reflective awareness," or *swadhyaya*, the fourth inner observance. The turning of awareness inward reminds us again and again that the inner life we are seeking is as close as our nose. Finally, we can live as an expression of all these attitudes when we celebrate the fact of our aliveness and surrender to life and to God (*ishvarapranidhana*).

We use the practice of Yoga, not to correct or punish ourselves for who we are not, but to see who we actually are. Yogis saw the illusion of disconnection as the true original sin because this misunderstanding causes us to live in a way that belies our fundamental goodness. In the yogic view we are thus born with original blessing—in essence, born divine.

Our true nature, however, is quite different from and often contradictory to what we call human nature. Certainly at times it is hard to believe in the basic goodness of a true nature—our own or others'. How could these *yamas* and *niyamas* possibly be a reflection of who we really are when people do such terrible things to each other? How could our true nature be one of peacefulness and compassion when, observing our everyday thoughts, we find ourselves entrenched in negativity and destructive emotions? Patanjali tells us that the failure to recognize our intrinsic goodness is caused by a momentary inability to perceive the silent and omnipresent life living itself through us. And why do we not perceive this silent and fundamentally benign backdrop? For the most part our primary modus operandi consists of identifying with and participating in the transitory movement of thoughts, feelings, memories, fantasies, and sensations and our ideas and judgments about ourselves and others. This veritable extravaganza of sensations is so compelling and so interesting, and so seemingly real, that we start to believe that this is who we really are. The dramatic enactment of these passing phenomena eclipses our view into our core self. We may believe that we are our anger, our pain, or our disappointment. We may be convinced that we are only our body, our wrinkles, or our successes or failures. When we get beneath all these exterior embellishments, we discover, as my elderly friend Denis tells me, looking down at his weathered hands, that we are "just the same person" in a different body. Through practice we emphatically prove that the parading sensations and identities that we may have found so convincing are actually temporary visitors, and when we become quiet and focused enough we understand that in hosting these visitors, our house, the Self, remains unchanged. Or as Patanjali describes in the very first sutras that define Yoga:

Yoga is the settling of the mind into silence.
When the mind has settled, we are established in our essential
    nature, which is unbounded Consciousness.

But immediately following these verses we're given the bad news that for the most part,

Our essential nature is usually overshadowed by the activity of the mind.[5]

What we are to practice, then, is an active inquiry into the nature of our true being. Because our false identity has been created through the ministrations of our habitual mind, we cannot solve a problem with the same mind that created it. Therefore, we have to change our mind. If you have ever had an argument with a loved one and found yourself and your beloved proceeding along a well-worn track that will lead to one or the other of you slamming a door, you know that as long as each of you holds to a point of view, nothing can change. Thus it is not until we are able to change our point of view that we can consider an alternative to the limited life we may be leading.

To wed the mind to its essence, we have to resist our habit of see-ing ourselves as separate. Tibetans have a saying: "Engaging in vir-tuous practice is as hard as pulling a tired donkey up a hill, but engaging in negative, destructive activities is as easy as rolling a boul-der down a steep slope."[6] At first this might appear to contradict the premise that we are fundamentally good, yet it does not. It is our ten-dency to see ourselves as separate, not an intrinsically horrible nature, that causes us to act out in destructive ways. It is this same tendency that causes schoolchildren, some as young as six or seven, to shoot their classmates or teachers because they have stopped seeing these people as human beings and instead see them as faceless enemies lack-ing in feelings. Anyone who has ever been overwhelmed by the emo-tions of anger, hatred, or jealousy will be familiar with the fierce struggle that takes place to resist acting in a way that is as destructive to our own well-being as to others. Yet as we consistently swim against the current of our habitual nature, we find ourselves moving into a gentler stream: we cause less harm, we invite less harm. That this swimming against the current is not easy helps explain why

Patanjali tells us everything we need to know about Yoga in the very first four Yoga sutras and then proceeds with 192 more, as if to say, "In case you didn't understand what I meant, here are 192 to clarify what I just said!" It is likely that we will not and cannot understand what Patanjali is talking about in those first revelatory sutras because our reading of his treatise will be filtered through the distorted lens of our habitual mind. We cannot understand this unbounded consciousness with a mind that is entangled in the false conditioning of separateness. So he gives us a very practical solution. He tells us to practice the ten noble qualities: be truthful, be peaceful, be selfless, be aware, be open, be generous, and be still. Only then we will come to realize that this is who we actually are. No matter how difficult it is to practice these virtues, in the final analysis we prevent ourselves from unnecessary suffering by practicing them. And, with a compassion that could have been born only from the experience of one who had also struggled, Patanjali gives us hundreds of practices for revealing these noble qualities.

What do we have to gain through practicing these ten precepts? Patanjali make a series of astute assessments that offer great hope and optimism about our choice to live in a gentler way. These sutras tell us what we will gain through allowing our ten noble qualities to shine forth. These dialectical sutras reveal that the very practice we avoid for fear of losing something delineates astonishing gains. In a world where we are schooled to take care of Number One, these verses systematically demolish some of the most deeply held mores of our culture.

> When one perseveres in nonviolence, hostility vanishes in its
>   presence. (2.35)
> Through the devoted practice of not taking things, the greatest
>   treasures are made manifest. (2.37)
> At its best, moderation produces the highest individual vitality.
>   (2.38)
> From contentment, unsurpassed happiness is gained. (2.42)[7]

That our own encumbered mind or our despair that things could be any different might prevent us from seeing these possibilities should not prevent us from trying. Patanjali doesn't ask us to go on blind faith: he beckons us to practice and prove these observations sound in the face of our own direct experience. This we can do in the testing ground of everyday life.

The *yamas* and *niyamas* are given as uncompromising, universal truths to be practiced regardless of our race, country, class, or circumstance. I well remember a teacher giving a talk about the *yama* of nonviolence *(ahimsa)* and saying that each time we kick someone out of our heart we develop a hole in our self and that hole cannot be repaired until we invite this person back in. My first response was: "What a lovely thought!" But almost instantaneously I rallied: "There has to be a footnote to this law! There must be some fine print at the bottom that says except your mother-in-law or that horrible colleague who gossips or the estranged friend who betrayed me." And then it became clear—the degree to which there are exceptions is the degree to which the mind still holds to its old point of view. This is why Yoga practice involves such a methodical and painstaking examination of where we have created convenient loopholes for ourselves. This is why working with our most deeply held resentments and grudges can bring about the greatest change, because it is here that we start to deconstruct the scaffolding upon which all our other points of view are based.

Through systematically deconstructing these false notions, we naturally begin to think and act from a place of goodness. This natural goodness is fundamentally different from "being good," which implies effort and self-coercion. When we view the world from a perspective of connectedness, acting from our higher nature becomes our most likely choice. We don't have to struggle to be these higher qualities. What we undoubtedly *will* struggle to do, however, is to change our point of view. Coming to the place where we are able to see from this new vantage point is the radical process of transmutation that Patanjali has in mind for us.

Yoga is not a spiritual practice for those who wish to be spectators on the field of life. Neither is it a practice for those given to dry intellectual speculation. It is not a practice to be applied only with people who agree with us or people we like. Yoga is an ongoing participatory experiment in which the world and every part of our life becomes our laboratory. It is a hands-on practice that can work only with our fullest and most complete participation at all times, every minute of the day, every day of the year, from our first breath to our last. It is this active inquiry that will gradually change our point of view. We will undoubtedly discover that what we take to be our "normal" state of being, and what we defend and tenaciously cling to, is the very source of our misery. This suffering is self-generated, and by the same logic, we are the only ones who can generate our own inner freedom.

Although Patanjali describes many extraordinary powers and supreme states of consciousness that can come through the practice of Yoga, these are not the primary concern of this book. Neither am I interested in metaphysical speculation on the difference between one form of *samadhi* or another. The world is not in dire need of people who can be in two places at one time or who can suspend themselves in hyperconscious states while living in a cave. But the world *is* in terrible need of greater kindness, generosity, and wisdom. These capacities are well within the reach of anyone willing to devote himself or herself sincerely to practice.

In this active inquiry into the nature of our true being, it is irrelevant what tradition, form, or style of Yoga we practice and whether we manage to touch our feet to the back of our head as a result. How we practice and whether our Yoga involves *asana, pranayama,* prayer, meditation, chanting, devotion, study, or altruistic work is of no great import. The best practice can only be defined as the one that works. What matters is that whatever we do we hold to the intention and spirit of the practice, which is to bring together rather than to pull apart. If our practice cultivates superiority and divisiveness, as it so often does between those practicing different religions and in variant

Yoga traditions, then we have clearly missed the point and purpose of practice.

As we shall see in chapter 4, we practice nothing more than becoming a human being. Learning to be a human being is a lifelong process. Yet we need not be great yogic scholars to understand the spirit of this practice. We need not learn Sanskrit or recite the list of *yamas* and *niyamas*, although it can be helpful to give each one careful thought and regular attention. Rather, we can regularly ask ourselves these questions: Who am I becoming through this practice? Am I becoming the world in which I wish to live?

Chapter 4

Yoga as a Life Practice

Perennial joy or passing pleasure?
This is the choice one is to make always.
The wise recognize these two, but not
The ignorant. The first welcome what leads
To abiding joy, though painful at the time.
The latter run, goaded by their senses,
After what seems immediate pleasure.

The first leads one to Self-realization:
The second makes one more and more
Estranged from his real Self.

KATHA UPANISHAD 2.2–2.4
Translated by Eknath Easwaran

A spiritual seeker with a penchant for philosophical speculation went traveling in search of wisdom. Coming upon some yogis lying naked on a huge rock in the broiling midday sun, he was immediately impressed by this austerity and hurried to the nearby village to find out who these people were. He discovered the sadhus were the bearers of profound wisdom and were capable of remarkable feats. Excited by his findings, he ran back to the group still sweltering under the sun. "I have come seeking knowledge and wish to discuss the nature of the universe with you," he said. "We'd be glad to," they replied, "as soon as you take your clothes off and get down on this rock."[1]

The word *Yoga* describes both a state of purified perception and the practices associated with attaining this clear way of seeing. The two meanings of the word give us some insight into the intimate link between the effort required to attain understanding and the imminence of realizing that which is already present within us. Today it is unlikely that we will be called to perform austerities under the hot sun, but there is no denying the necessarily practical nature of Yoga. As with all things, there is no free lunch. The sixteenth-century treatise Yoga-Sara-Samgraha ("Compendium on the Essence of Yoga") makes a distinction between aspirants who "think" about and would like a spiritual life *(arurukshu)* and those who are actually practicing *(yunjana)*. This succinct categorization tells us that not much has changed in human nature since time immemorial. There is yet a third category of aspirant: those who, through consistent practice, have become steady in their wisdom *(Yoga-arudha, yukta-* or *sthita-prajna).*[2] Patanjali tells us unequivocally that while there are rare instances of spontaneous realization, the great majority of us will come to this clear way of seeing over a lifetime of consistent practice. If this, as one of my students bemoaned, "feels like a life sentence," we might ask, what better way is there to spend the rest of our lives? Ironically, most of us already unconsciously invest a great deal of our time and energy in pursuits that lead to our own and others' suffering. This very same energy, this same time, when redirected can bring about a movement toward peacefulness. Whenever we practice, with every breath and attempt to focus the mind, the goal of Yoga is in a sense already realized. It is as immediate as that.

In this book I use the terms *life practice* and *spiritual practice* interchangeably. Unfortunately, the word *spiritual* has come to imply an inherent dualism in which everyday life is made to look paltry and mundane in stark contrast to the imagined heavenly realms to which we can only aspire. For most of us this ideal realm seems terribly vague and elusive, especially when juxtaposed with the all-too-real and encumbering nature of life on earth. The word *spiritual* seems to conjure up images of ethereal worlds, billowing clouds, and a pie-in-the-sky realm where everyone is always smiling and nice to each other. Because most of us would have to walk a long road to find such a place, having a spiritual life can seem strangely alienating. But more important, if we have to go somewhere else to have a spiritual life, what about the life we leave behind?

Thus I call the practice of Yoga a life practice. By *life practice* I mean an ongoing inquiry into how to be completely engaged and intimate with the wild force that runs through everything and is running through us, if we would but pause long enough to notice. A life practice, then, is anything that we do over an extended period of time that consistently and reliably deepens the connection to our experience and expression of aliveness. While Yoga offers us a vast repertoire of formal practices that accommodate the different predilections of individuals, almost any activity can be used as a life practice if it reconnects us with the source of our aliveness. There is no comprehending the wily ways of the daimon, who lures us to paint, to sing, to dance, compose music, build sanctuaries, plant gardens, raise children, write poetry, climb mountains, and do all of the other things humans do to discover themselves in life. All such activities, if practiced mindfully and with passionate devotion, can be called a form of Yoga. The greater purpose of a formal Yoga practice, however, is to apply the acute attentiveness we learn on the mat to all aspects of our everyday life so that this unitive awareness filters through our relationships, our work, and our play. If our formal practice fails to translate in this way, it has failed us utterly. By anchoring our spiritual practice always within everyday life, we remove the arbitrary barriers between what is considered spiritual and extraordinary and what is material and ordinary.

By *life practice* I also mean any activity or attitude that helps us have a direct experience of the shimmering life force that stands behind and suffuses all things. Through such a practice we come to know that the most reliable and consistent thing about us *is* the silent substratum that lies beneath all passing and changing phenomena. In Yoga we create a situation in which relaxing into life becomes more likely to occur. This deliberate and intentional creating of a context in which we explore the invisible, magical, and mysterious is the basis of all true and authentic Yoga practice. Very simply, we set aside time and a quiet place to engage in inquiries that will remind us of who we really are. We do this practice as often as necessary for this understanding to become an implicit part of our being. For most of us this means practicing from the first breath to the last.

At the same time, a life practice must help us to find a practical relationship with the dynamic and unpredictable aspects of our life. We establish a calm abiding center, not to fortify ourselves against the chaos of life, but to help us become resilient, tolerant, and accepting of the inevitable, perplexing, and often agonizing losses we all go through. A calm abiding center and a fully engaged life, therefore, go hand in hand. This inner tempering through the fire of practice allows us to live at higher and higher levels of charge: to feel intensely, love intensely, and work intensely without fracturing in the process. We make firm this abiding center of equanimity, but not to sequester ourselves from life or to make life less "lively." Rather, as the photographer Henri Cartier-Bresson once said about capturing life through the lens of his camera, we "discipline reality." Cartier-Bresson did not lessen the poignancy of his subject matter through being attentive to it. In the same way, when we practice Yoga we do not dampen the fiery nature of life: if anything, we place ourselves right in the fierce heat of the center.

One of the simplest ways we can make firm our desire to practice Yoga is to choose a particular place for our formal practice and, if possible, a particular time each day to visit this place. While having an extra room in the house to devote solely to practice is fortunate, it is not necessary. A small area in your bedroom or living room will work perfectly well if you can have privacy and quiet during the time you are practicing. If you work at home, make sure your practice place is far enough from your office to give you the necessary mental distance from the distractions of work.

Just as a church, temple, or synagogue develops a palpable air of serenity and calm, your practice place, over time, can become your own personal sanctuary. Make sure that you keep this place clean and fresh and regularly clear the space of any distracting paraphernalia that may have accumulated. You may want to create a small altar or focal point for your practice space, where you can light a candle, place a fresh flower daily, or have pictures of your family members, teachers, or articles that have meaning for you. You might also want to place on it pictures of people who are ill or suffering whom you wish to hold in your heart. Make a point of attending to this focal point each day, brushing away the ash of old incense, dusting the objects clean, and otherwise beginning each practice in a gesture of renewal and focused attention.

Have all your Yoga equipment, whether that is a mat and a meditation cushion or a retinue of Yoga props and accessories, neatly stored and ready at hand. If possible, do not use these things for any other purpose. A Yoga blanket covered with cracker crumbs or dog hair is not likely to inspire your practice. When you assign a single purpose to the place and the objects in it, gradually your practice space will become sacred.

Each time you visit your practice space, make a deliberate attempt to secure your peace and quiet during this time: let the answering machine take your calls, let other householders know you do not wish to be disturbed, and otherwise reinforce your intention to focus your attention inward. If you live with others, you may need to schedule your practice early in the morning before the rest of the household is in full swing. If private time runs counter to your responsibilities, as is often the case for parents with young children, graciously welcome your infants and children into the practice, integrating as best you can your duty to those in your care and your commitment to yourself. Children and animals are particularly sensitive to their environment and will often join in a practice in a spirit of playfulness and curiosity, becoming quiet as a practice session continues. I have watched children who really enjoy being with their parents during practice time, even if only to fall asleep nestled in their parent's lap while the adult meditates.

While it is helpful to minimize distractions, this should not be at the expense of the greater integrity of your life, and it cannot be achieved by blocking them out. The phone ringing, the neighbor's dog barking, the repair person who arrives just as you are settling in: these are all opportunities to stay centered in the midst of everyday life. Simply note these momentary distractions, attend to them if you must, and return to your practice. Or if this is not possible, let the task or the distraction *become* your practice: listening to a distraught friend, tending a sick child, driving one's mother to the doctor. If you have many tasks to juggle, as I do, keep a notepad next to your practice mat, and if you have an idea, a thought, or an errand that needs remembering, jot it down and then return to your practice.

The purpose of a formal practice time is to establish and sustain the awareness of inner tranquillity that is always available to us. In the hubbub of everyday life it is easy to forget that each of us has this innate capacity to be calm and peaceful. In our formal practice time we try to create the ideal hothouse conditions for cultivating a strong connection with our center. Ultimately, we can draw no definitive line between formal practice and everyday life. However, a word of caution to those who assert there is no need for formal practice since the whole of their life is practice: I know of no sincere or authentic practitioners who claim to be so mature in their understanding that practice has become unnecessary.

When you finish with your practice, put everything away. Fold your blankets neatly and clear the space. This final gesture will ensure that when you return to your practice space you can make a fresh beginning.

Daily practice provides a context in which we can gradually awaken to ourselves as we are. Daily practice should not be construed as a chronological progression toward a new and improved self, or our practice time will be fraught with subtle self-aggression. Water and ice are of the same substance but of different freedoms. As soon as you sit or make your breath smooth and even or remain quiet within a Yoga posture, you are already realizing the goal of Yoga: inner stillness. This inner stillness is as imminent as your focus.

While the practices of Yoga do indeed involve discipline, will-power, determination, and great effort, the experience of Yoga happens spontaneously. This may seem at first a contradiction in terms, but it is not. A musician may train for years, practicing scales, developing fluency, and studying the masters, but it is not until the musician can go beyond effort and let go of everything known that an alchemical transformation can take place. When the musician's skill has become so much a part of his or her being that there is no separation between the musician, the instrument, and the music, then the art of music happens. Yoga is thus not something we can make happen but something that *happens to us.* But it does not happen by accident.

That Yoga is not serendipitous is good news. How then do we make ourselves more prone to this happening? Quite simply, we develop mastery by doing what all the great spiritual masters did. No one was ever cured of an illness simply through reading medical journals, and in the same way no one ever realized Yoga through simply rubbing shoulders with a great guru or through intellectual speculation on scriptures and texts. Even Christ and Buddha were ordinary people when they were born. Consider the thousands of people who had contact with these great teachers but remained ignorant. We become the consciousness of Christ or Buddha or Krishna through doing what they did. There is nothing elusive about Yoga—except we tend to avoid what is obvious under the misguided notion that it might be better (and more enjoyable) to sit back and wait for some good luck to come our way.

Doing the practices of an adept are rarely easy. In the epic battle told in the Bhagavad Gita, Arjuna faces his fear of entering into a fight in which he must slay his friends and relatives. Yet Arjuna's battle is not so different from the challenges and ethical dilemmas we face each day: keeping our cool with our children, staying centered in bumper-to-bumper traffic, or coping with uncertainty when our workplace undergoes a downsizing. Through practice we undermine such fears.

Krishna's advice to Arjuna could well be our own:

On this path effort never goes to waste,
and there is no failure. Even a little effort
toward spiritual awareness will protect you
from the greatest fear. (2:40)[3]

When we begin Yoga practice in earnest, we are signing up for a lifelong apprenticeship with our Self and to the Self. And as in any apprenticeship, many skills can be learned only over a long period of time. There are no shortcuts and no crash courses, and there is no replacement for the satisfaction and richness that follow in the wake of such wholehearted commitment. The very idea of a lifelong apprenticeship has become quite foreign in our culture, invested as it is in securing immediate benefits as a wedge against uncertainty. In my own lengthy apprenticeship as a student teacher, I learned from watching my mentor Yoga teacher and physical therapist, Judith Lasater, work with people over the course of many years. I watched how she worked with people on the first day of Yoga class and how she worked with the same person many years later. This gave me crucial insights into the nature of the human mind and the complexity of the body, insights that could not be replicated over a weekend. I like to tell my own teacher trainees that Yoga is not Woodworking 101 but Japanese carpentry. Our teachers may show us precisely how to bevel the edge of a table or chair, but there is only one person who can bevel that edge. No matter how clear the teacher's description or careful her demonstration, it may still take a hundred crooked, crude, and rough attempts to become proficient and produce that smooth edge. Just as a poorly sanded surface will splinter fingers for years to come, false understanding will continually sabotage a life. What we produce through such patient artistry is a spiritual understanding of enduring beauty.

We may find that when we begin our practice we have a low tolerance for frustration. We may use any slipup as evidence that we have unwisely placed our faith in such a practice. Through our cultural conditioning, we may falsely believe that things *should* come easily, that life should be as it is on TV: a series of climactic moments where everyone is having a birthday. Or we blame someone else: "If the teacher were clearer, I'm sure I would get this." But nothing can replace the minutes, hours, and days of practice, observation, and just plain old trial and error involved in a lifelong apprenticeship. It is the very slowness of this apprenticeship that *is* the healing, for in slowing down we fall into a more natural rhythm with life and with ourselves. Thus we gradually change, gradually understand, gradually integrate the unconscious material of the psyche into the conscious mind, and the incremental nature of these changes ensures that we metamorphose without losing anything in the equation.

In parts of the English countryside one can see amazing stone walls, fashioned from rocks of all sizes and dimensions. Many of these walls consist of stones that have been removed from the pastures, thereby improving the grazing land. It surely would have been quicker to throw the stones in a heap, but even after a short time such a wall would begin to disintegrate and, when tested, give way to marauding livestock. Many of these walls have no mortar but are held together by the careful placement of stones with complementary shapes. Making such a wall must have taken considerable thought and patience. This perfect fit has given the walls their solidity, durability, and beauty. In the same way, time acts as an invisible mortar for our experience; it is what stands between potentially discordant elements and, through finding their correct relationship, brings all into a unified whole.

If this all sounds like a rough deal, we might consider being grateful to our spiritual ancestors that instead of selling us a snake oil remedy they were honest enough to let us know that the cure for what ails us might take a lifetime. We might take heart in the fact that thousands of years ago wise people called seers (because their process of seeing was so clear that they saw the true nature of things) observed natural phenomena and came to some startling conclusions about what happens when our minds cease to be limited by the false understanding of division. But at the same time, they made one mundane and pragmatic recommendation after another about how to gain a truthful understanding of ourselves. These seers also made lists of the umpteen ways we delude ourselves and the umpteen roadblocks and distractions we are likely to encounter during our apprenticeship, which we'll look at in detail in later chapters. Instead of being discouraged by their conclusions, we can be heartened that, just like us, thousands of years ago, there were people who had a hard time getting out of bed in the morning. People who ate too much, lacked faith and willpower, and who, if they did "get it," forgot what they'd learned. We can take heart in the fact that our spiritual ancestors floundered just as we do and were kind enough to document the highlights and the pitfalls of their journey to aid us. We might also develop a sense of humor so that we can laugh at ourselves when we fall down and take our shambling efforts, not as a sign of personal failure, but as proof of the authenticity of our endeavor. We would be wise, then, to be wary of any methodology (whether it be a diet plan or a tidy-up-your-life plan) that promises immediate results and all-conclusive, happily-ever-after guarantees.

Lest this give the impression that a life practice such as Yoga is a somber and unpleasant undertaking akin to a daily dose of nasty-tasting medicine, let me say that I intend neither to glorify or to cover up the often difficult nature of such a path. In the Bhagavad Gita Krishna advises Arjuna that such a path seems like poison at first but tastes like nectar in the end, and that which tastes like nectar at first is often bitter poison in the end (18.37–39).[4] We may assume a false sense of liberty and feel an initial resistance to putting reins on a life that we believe to be free. Yet this false sense of freedom almost always moves us further away from our true self and from real happiness.

What we shall discover is that the practice *is* the reward. The moment we sit in quiet self-reflection, slowly stretch our limbs, or enter deep relaxation, we become the thing that we are seeking, and in doing so it is possible to experience the end result from the very beginning. Anyone who has ever planted and tended a garden knows there is as much pleasure in digging a hole for a sapling as there is in admiring the full-grown tree. The very thought that someone will admire this tree long after we've died can give us satisfaction in the moment. Whether we're pulling weeds from a flower bed, harvesting fruit, or shoveling manure to make compost, it doesn't take a fait accompli garden paradise to bring about happiness.

Of all the qualities that can transform a life practice, gratitude and faith stand supreme. The supporting qualities of these two noble attributes transform every aspect of practice from start to finish. Before you begin your Yoga practice, spend a few moments contemplating these truths. First you are alive. You happened! It could well have turned out differently. Second, your life circumstances are such that you could afford to buy this book, and you are educated enough to read it. It is likely that you have shelter, a place to sleep, and food to eat. Further, you have access to spiritual teachings, teachers, and the time to practice. These are indications of extraordinary good fortune. Those who find themselves in such favorable circumstances are only a fraction of the world's people. Recognizing these facts and contemplating their significance is a good way to start the day, helping to erase cynicism and bringing a freshness to each new day. No matter how sore, tired, or unwell you feel, what incredible good fortune that you have the tools to improve your condition and your life.

Recognizing this good fortune turns the most difficult circumstance on its head. Instead of, "Woe is me, my back hurts," we can say, "Isn't it fortunate I have some tools to alleviate my pain." Instead of "My life is so hard right now," we can affirm, "What a blessing to have a practice to get me through this tough time." If you are new to practice you may find these affirmations a stretch, but those of you who have a lifetime of practice behind you will remember the many difficult times when the only thing that got you through was your spiritual practice. Many people do not have the support of such a practice, and even if life is terribly difficult, it is likely that your circumstances will be better than others' just by the fact that you have been drawn to a spiritual quest.

You may wish to contemplate the hundreds of teachers and thousands of practitioners who have kept this tradition alive over the centuries, sometimes at great sacrifice. When I imagine all these ancestral teachers, and the ones of my own lifetime, I feel incredibly lucky to have received such a rich inheritance. Begin your practice with a prayer of intent to use these teachings wisely and never to take them for granted.

When this feeling of gratitude begins to build, it will naturally generate a faith in your practice, the purpose of your life, and your own abilities. Gratitude and faith go together, hand in hand. When I meet people who do not realize how fortunate they are to receive teachings, I feel very sad. They are not able to recognize the priceless value of the teachings, and this jaded attitude impedes any real learning. This lack of recognition affects them not only in a Yoga class, but in every waking hour of their day. If we can't appreciate the beauty of something as wonderful as Yoga, how can we appreciate the warm bed, the hot running water, and the people who care for us?

So before you begin your practice, take a moment to reflect on your exceptional circumstances. Without this gratitude, no matter what you practice—on your mat or meditation cushion—you will always be a little sour inside. With it, the very same practice takes on a sweetness and that sweetness lingers throughout the day. There is something very tender about this gratitude: through it we recognize that life itself, without adornment or elaboration, is a gift. Simplifying things in this way, we can foster gratitude regardless of our circumstances. In the spirit of this gratefulness, let your practice begin.

Part 2

On the Means

Chapter 5

Slowing Down

*Our perception that we have "no time" is one of the distinctive marks
of modern Western culture.*
Margaret Visser

*When science finally locates the center of the universe, some people will
be surprised to discover that they're not in it.*
Source unknown

Slowing down is the precursor to Yoga practice because this simple act
allows us to consider our thoughts, feelings, and actions more carefully
in the light of our desire to live peacefully. When we overwork, when
we try to fit too many things into an already congested schedule, when
we rush from place to place, we lose track of what is important, and in
doing so we almost always fail to serve those values that support our
relationships and our heartfelt aspirations. A certain harshness can
creep into our interactions with others, and this is the same harshness
we ourselves find so distressing and so undermining of our sense of
connectedness. We can become curt with our friends, family, and co-
workers in a way that belies their importance to us. Maybe we become
so exhausted by all our busyness that we're irritable when we wish to be
kind, thoughtless when we want our actions to be considerate. So before we sink our teeth into the foundations of Yoga practice, consider
this one possibility: that you have all the time you need. When you
find yourself rushing, you can catch yourself and breathe out fully, af-
firming that you do indeed have all the time you need. You can ask
yourself if the sky will fall down, if someone will die, or if the world
will stop spinning if you sit down for ten minutes and breathe the air.

When we slow down we create a conducive environment for kindness and thoughtfulness to flourish. We find that it isn't necessary to join our local peace demonstration. We can demonstrate for peace by being peaceful. We can take the time to chat with our elderly neighbor and demonstrate through our bearing what our values are.

When we slow down we make a place for silence and solitude in our lives. There need be nothing complicated or austere about either of these practices; they are a natural component of any day lived at a human pace. One of my more recent spiritual teachers is a man called Ernie, who probably has never read a spiritual book or sat on a meditation cushion in his life. "All you crazy people," he tells me, "rushing around doing big things. All you need is a little space out in nature. Heals most things, I reckon." A day with Ernie is a day spent with a master: he doesn't say much, but when he does it is always an incisive observation. Sitting on the grass having lunch with Ernie, you notice an air of stillness around him—he's just so pleased to be alive (now almost seventy), taking in the day, listening to the birds, enjoying the fresh clean air. "My, that sun does feel good," he says. And neither is Ernie a couch potato; he can walk over a property and assess the most urgent tasks: this gate needs resetting, those thistles need cutting. "I'd remove that barbed wire if I were you," he tells me. And then without any fanfare, Ernie shows up with his tools, sun hat, socks, and sandals and accomplishes, at a remarkably slow pace, more than most of us could do in a week. Striking up a conversation with the local farmers, I can feel myself start to get edgy: there's work to do, and this rambling chitchat doesn't seem to be serving a purpose. After we turn back to work, Ernie has noted all the valuable information that has just been exchanged: "Told me exactly the species of oak that will thrive in this soil." Over tea, he casually remarks, "Good neighbors are mighty important. Never any time wasted making friends for yourself."

Most of us could learn more from spending a day with Ernie than a month in India sitting in a cave. In Yoga practice we set up Ernie-like conditions in a more deliberate way, but there need be nothing contrived about making room for more quiet inward time. Although spending some time each day in formal solitary practice is helpful, we can practice an inward solitude, as Ernie has taught me, even when we're in company. By not talking so much, we automatically create more silent spaces in between things. By not doing so much, we create natural pauses to reflect. By not spreading ourselves thin doing things that aren't that important, we open up time for the things that are.

You can anchor your desire to slow down by finding one thing in your life that defines this more natural rhythm. For instance, I decided many years ago that it was a basic necessity to cook one good meal every day and take the time to enjoy it, by myself or with others. If I don't have time for that one meal, there's something amiss with my life and I adjust accordingly. Maybe for you it's having the time to read a story to your child or walking the dog or spending part of the weekend tending your roses. Perhaps it's having the time to cuddle with your partner and share the events of the day before you go to sleep. The degree to which you do not believe you have time to spend even ten minutes sitting quietly is the degree to which you desperately need to spend ten minutes sitting quietly. If we did nothing else in our spiritual practice but reduce our accelerated pace, the world would be transformed overnight.

When we find ourselves hurrying or pressing others out of our way, we might ask ourselves exactly where we are going in such a rush. What are we running away from, and what are we running toward? Pause for moment. Sit down and relax. Smell the air. Look around you. Take a deep breath in and out. This state of mind called Yoga can't be found anywhere else but here. The moment opens itself for you. Will you step in?

Chapter 6

Cleaning Up Our Act:
The Four *Brahmavihara*

Those who see all beings in themselves,
And themselves in all beings,
Relinquish hatred.
How can the seeming diversity of life
Delude the one who has seen its unity?

ISHA UPANISHAD 6–7
Translated by Donna Farhi

Descriptions of the enlightened state abound in spiritual literature, and as resplendent and inspiring as these descriptions are, when we are drowning they are about as useful to us as a swimming manual. What we need at these moments is something that can help us keep our head above water. Patanjali tells us that we are drowning because of one fundamental misunderstanding: we fail to see who we are, and so we live in a state of mistaken identity. As with a character in a comedic drama, our life as an impostor becomes ever more entangled and complicated until we are able to realize and live as our true identity: we are not an island unto ourselves but inextricably linked to everyone and everything. Because our suffering arises out of the conviction of our separateness, until we change our point of view all our strategies are as effective as changing deck chairs on the *Titanic*. But Patanjali was also a pragmatist and saw nothing wrong with changing deck chairs, if indeed these intermediary measures gradually led to a changed point of view. He understood so well the common ways in which we flounder that he gave compassionate suggestions to ameliorate our suffering. These suggestions are not merely stopgap measures; instead, they gradually build a foundation for a new way of experiencing ourselves.

Patanjali was so familiar with the obstacles to happiness and mental clarity that he made concise lists of the causes of suffering and self-torment, known as *kleshas,* as well as useful suggestions for overcoming them. While the Yoga-Sutra is liberally spiced with handy hints for overcoming these *kleshas,* Patanjali returns again and again to describe the enlightened state like a composer using a refrain to anchor the central melody in our minds. Go ahead and whittle away at these obstacles, he tells us, but know that your happiness depends on seeing one true thing—who you really are. Recognizing your true self will irrevocably transform your every thought and action. The enlightened yet physically deformed sage Ashtavakra derided the king's spiritual aides for failing to see beyond his physical form to the infinite nature that lay beneath it. When King Janaka saw that the courtiers he had surrounded himself with were but fools in light of Ashtavakra's wisdom, he asked Ashtavakra to be his teacher. In one of the first of many dialogues recorded in the Ashtavakra Gita, Ashtavakra tells the king:

> If you detach yourself from the identification
> with the body and remain relaxed in and as
> Consciousness, you will, this very moment,
> be happy, at peace, free from bondage.[1]

But then, like Patanjali, Ashtavakra continues with hundreds of other teaching verses, aware that such a realization can come only when we have utterly surrendered to a different point of view. Like the classic joke of the city slicker asking the farmer for directions, only to be told, "You can't get there from here," we can't get there from our present perspective. So Patanjali gives us some homework to do, and every now and again asks the question: "Do you see it now?" And because it is likely that we don't yet see clearly, or we see partially or through a smudge on the lens of perception, he gives us more homework to do.

Patanjali lists the five causes of suffering, or *kleshas*, as:

1. *Avidha:* Ignorance of our eternal nature
2. *Asmita:* Seeing oneself as separate and divided from the rest of the world
3. *Raga:* Attraction and attachment to impermanent things
4. *Dvesha:* Aversion to the unpleasant
5. *Abhinivesha:* Clinging to life because we fail to perceive the seamless continuity of consciousness, which cannot be broken by death (Yoga-Sutra 2.3)

All the other *kleshas* are born out of the first, *avidha*, or "not seeing." The *kleshas* exist within us in various states of latency or arousal. We might think we're getting our act together, then someone pushes our buttons, triggering a habitual and overblown reaction. The degree to which our reactions are inappropriate is usually the degree to which a *klesha* holds sway. And the degree to which we defend our reaction is usually a strong indicator that we are in the vicinity of our personal blind spot. This misunderstanding has become so much a part of our identity that, like the nose on our face, we have trouble seeing it. So how do we remove these obstructions to clear seeing? Patanjali goes on to tell us there are nine obstacles to mental clarity. They are lack of effort, fatigue or disease, dullness or inertia, doubt, carelessness, laziness or sloth (habitual disinclination toward exertion), inability to turn attention inward, perverted or distorted seeing, inability to establish a firm ground for practice (lack of perseverance), and inability to sustain a firm ground for practice (regression). The presence of a sorrowful mood, depression, frustration, psychological despair, physical restlessness, and rough, restricted breathing are all strong indicators that the mind is disturbed by these obstacles (Yoga-Sutra 1.30, 31).

In part 3 we'll look at many of these obstacles in detail. Most of us are all too aware of these obstacles, and when we see them in such a comprehensive list we may start shifting in our seats. The obstacles may appear too numerous or too overwhelming. We may feel so beleaguered by one, many, or all of them that we don't know where to begin. This is where Patanjali demonstrates enormous compassion. Although he suggests many practices, from breathing exercises to meditative techniques, he precedes all these suggestions with four down-to-earth recommendations. They are presented as prerequisites to clearing the mind, and, as we shall see, their practice has a domino effect on removing the other obstacles. These four recommendations represent the kingpin: knock this pin over, and all the others will topple too.

Surprisingly, we are not told to find ourselves a nice little secluded cave in which to begin our practice. Rather, we are advised to begin our practice by cleaning up our social relationships. He suggests that we develop four attitudes (*brahmavihara*) to life's challenges and apply these to all our relationships and in all situations. These qualities of the heart are conducive to peace of mind and thus can enable us to overcome the distractions that already exist in the mind and to prevent the production of more psychological distress. They are:

1. Friendliness toward the joyful
2. Compassion for those who are suffering
3. Celebrating the good in others
4. Remaining impartial to the faults and imperfections of others
   (Yoga-Sutra I.33)

Our spiritual fitness can be tested only in relationship to others. We may ascribe to ourselves all kinds of spiritual attainments while we are perched on our meditation cushion, but do these attainments hold up when challenged in relationship? Are we like the dog that behaves nicely when patted and turns into a ferocious snapping beast the moment its fur is rubbed the wrong way? Testing these four attitudes in all our relationships can thus show us with great accuracy our present state of mind and our level of conditioning. But more

important, putting these *brahmavihara* into practice in our everyday relationships gradually dismantles our resistance to seeing ourselves as
unified with life.

Because our relationships tend to generate the most perturbation,
the practice of the four *brahmavihara* is designed to undermine the
causative factors of mental unrest and make it easier to bring the
mind into a tranquil state. Every day we encounter people doing good
things, people doing bad things, people we like, people we dislike,
and people who are plain driving us crazy. As long as we are in the
world this is unlikely to change, so how can we change our attitude to
the predictable difficulty of relationships?

The first *brahmavihara* is perhaps the easiest, and that is simply to
extend our friendship toward people who are already pleasantly dis-
posed toward us. We can do this in very real terms—by extending assistance and support to our friends when they need us and by availing
ourselves of the same support. Without being indiscriminate, we can
assume friendliness toward others in our daily interactions and by
doing so wear away at the thickness of our skin. Clearly, it is easier to
be friendly with someone who likes us or someone we admire, so by
starting with an easy practice we gain confidence in our ability to live
compassionately.

The second *brahmavihara*, being compassionate toward those who
are in pain, also looks relatively easy. Yet so many of us have become
so distanced from suffering, or hardened and anesthetized by the
magnitude of it and our apparent impotence to do anything about it,
that we have to rediscover our empathetic capacity. Developing empathy involves breaking down the arbitrary division between what is
personal and what is universal. We can start with those forms of
compassion that feel most tangible to us. Perhaps we have children
and therefore we can imagine what it would be like to lose a child to
illness, by accident, or through violence. So when we hear about the
death of a child, we can pause for a moment and imagine that grief as
our own. I have a friend who spent many difficult years adapting to
her new life as an immigrant in a foreign country. When she read a

story about an African man being attacked by white supremacists in her community, she identified so strongly with his feeling of aloneness that she sent presents to him and his children to let him know he was welcome in her country. This act of kindness to a complete stranger gave this new immigrant the courage to start a program to educate people about cultural diversity. Similarly, another friend had always had a fear of having her possessions stolen and took great solace in her home as a sanctuary. When she read of a single father who came home from his Christmas vacation with his two young daughters to discover his entire house ransacked by vandals, she felt compelled to arrange a meeting to give him money to replace some of his possessions.

Clearly, we can express compassion at several different levels, but I believe that all acts of compassion, whether done in prayer, in thought, or in deed, are practical. For many of us there will be a preliminary step to expressing compassion. We may need to start by noticing how often we deflect or ignore not only the suffering of others but even the basic rights, needs, and feelings of others. During a retreat based in a university campus dormitory, the cleaning staff related to our retreatants how unappreciated they felt by both students and teachers during the school year. As we got to know these normally invisible people, we found they strongly supported our efforts to study Yoga. When we took the time to greet them by name and thank them for keeping our accommodations clean, many were stunned that we noticed their existence. One man related how the students at the end of the school term would deliberately leave their dormitories "in such a filthy state, you wonder how these kids were raised." Shaking his head in disgust, he went on, "When I clean the women's bathroom, I tell the girls I've got teenagers of my own and I wouldn't want them to be walking around naked in front of a stranger. I put a sign up so I can get the work done quickly, but some of them just look at me as if I'm not there and walk around naked anyway." When our retreat group put together a basket of goodies to thank the cleaning staff for their contribution to our retreat, many said they had never been thanked, let alone presented with a gift for their work. After a while this habit of pausing and considering the situation of the other becomes as natural to us as our habit of considering our own story.

The next level of compassion may be consciously setting time aside to meditate on the well-being of others (in Buddhist meditation this is called *metta*, or loving-kindness meditation, and like Patanjali's *brahmavihara*, it begins with self-compassion and is gradually extended to include all sentient beings). Meditation or prayer can be a way of seeding loving-kindness and practicing the more difficult forms of compassion (such as dispassion for our enemies) in the hothouse conditions of daily practice.

Gradually, as we become more comfortable with being intimate with the suffering of others, we may extend our compassion in more active ways. We don't have to become Mother Teresa. A simple gesture, like bringing a pot of soup to a sick friend or sending a card to someone who is having a hard time to let them know we are thinking of them, is also an active form of compassion. Gradually, compassion becomes less something we practice and more something that we are. While it is not always possible to make our compassion known in tangible ways, the important thing is to begin where you are and to practice at whatever level feels authentic for you.

I well remember the growing sense of frustration and annoyance at the homeless people I often found outside my apartment steps when I lived in San Francisco. Frequently they urinated in the entryways or left the steps littered with bottles and stacks of filthy garbage. I felt threatened by being asked for money and repulsed by the smell of unwashed bodies. After a while I became very fearful of ever looking a homeless person in the eye or even acknowledging a friendly hello. Then one morning I came upon a sad old man sitting on the steps who asked me for some money. I forced myself to take a good look at him and to meet his gaze and then reflexively walked away. But as I walked away, I could not shake the thought that this man looked like my father. Perhaps he was someone else's father. Perhaps he had been my father in a past life. Without thinking, I walked back to the steps and emptied my change purse in front of his widening eyes. After that day, I decided to work one night a week at a homeless shelter, as much to relieve my own sense of impotence as to help others.

Another way that we practice the second *brahmavihara* is that when we are feeling bad we can imagine all the others who might be feeling just the same way and extend them compassion. I'm not sure why I find this one of the most comforting and effective *brahmavihara* practices: there is something immensely reassuring about sharing suffering rather than sequestering it. We can start to see that this suffering is not "our" suffering but a universal suffering. Maybe we feel lonely and we feel hopeless that we will ever find companionship. It's likely that there are thousands of people right this instant who are feeling the same loneliness. When we drive past an elderly woman waiting at the bus stop, we might pause and reflect. Perhaps she has been widowed for many years, perhaps she eats all her meals alone and has no one to talk to. Maybe one day this will happen to us. It doesn't matter whether this is exactly the case, but it matters that we make a habit of considering our kinship with others. In this way we practice seeing everyone as a reflection of some part of ourselves.

The point of the second *brahmavihara* is to whittle away at our sense of personal ownership of suffering. This is another way of shaking the foundations of our conviction that there is an "I," a "me," an "us," and a "them." All of these designations form the scaffolding that supports our separateness. When we whittle away at these structures of separation, eventually the whole old way of thinking starts to crumble.

The third *brahmavihara*, seeing the good in others, can be practiced on many levels. When we practice seeing the good in others and focusing on their praiseworthy qualities, we choose to see the implicit divinity in each person. One of our greatest challenges in meditation is to cut through the constant chatter of thoughts, ideas, stories, dramas, fantasies, and judgments to see through to the untouched canvas behind these manifestations. When we try to see through the annoying faults, foibles, and idiosyncratic traits of another to that person's basic goodness, we are looking for that same untouched canvas. Anyone who has been in any kind of intimate relationship can attest to the difficulty of seeing this goodness in another, especially when we have seen another's imperfections up close. When we gain some impartiality toward these imperfections, we begin to free ourselves of the critical internal monologue that fills so much of our waking thought.

Another dimension of the third *brahmavihara* is celebrating the good fortune and prosperity of others in an unqualified way. If you have ever noted some kind of happiness in another and almost simultaneously felt pity for your own situation, you know how deeply instilled this habit of comparison can be. A business associate lands a successful contract and we immediately feel a sense of envy. Or someone else has more people in her Yoga class and we feel a growing disdain for her popularity. There is a bumper sticker that reads: "Please, God, if you can't make me thin, make everyone else fat." This tells us a great deal about the way our cultural mind operates, obsessed as it is with competition and one-upmanship. One only has to pick up the magazines strategically placed at the checkout counter to see the degree to which so many of us revel in the misfortunes of others, such is our fascination and insatiable appetite for reading about the failed marriages, careers, and weight-loss plans of celebrities. We're taught to perceive someone else's success as a threat to our own, so the only way we can get ahead is if someone else is left behind. We may even have formed the habit of gaining pleasure from seeing others fail merely because it makes us feel so much better about ourselves. It can be particularly insightful to notice how often we fail to celebrate the good things that happen to other people.

The third *brahmavihara* can also be practiced by cultivating association with peaceful people who have already achieved a high level of spiritual awareness. As one of my teachers, Baba Hari Dass, once advised, "If you want to learn about peace, spend time with peaceful people." Traditionally this association came through a guru, teacher, or through living with other renunciates within an ashram or school. These are all worthy possibilities, but we can find many opportunities closer to home. We may have a grandparent, an uncle, or a friend in whose presence we feel accepted. When we are in the company of such a spiritual friend we feel a safety that allows us to be unselfconscious and honest. We can augment the positive effect of this connection by holding the image of this person in our hearts and minds. We might place a photograph of this person on an alter in our home. Or, if we're Christian, we may naturally turn this devotion toward Christ. If we practice Buddhism, we can turn this devotion toward Buddha. This imaging can be literal such as placing a statue of the Buddha in a prominent place or a form of inner visualization.

The last *brahmavihara*, practicing impartiality or detachment toward those who have harmed us, is the black belt of all the *brahmavihara*. The Bible tells us to love our neighbors and also to love our enemies. G. K. Chesterton once famously added, "probably because generally they are the same people." If we analyze the content of most of our meditative excursions, we will probably find them filled with the dramatic reruns of arguments, standoffs, fights, and criticisms of our perceived enemies. And, as the old saying goes, there is nothing more time-consuming than having an enemy. Further analysis might reveal that the selection of reruns is limited so that we rewind, replay, and re-script our past and imagined future interactions with alarming regularity. We might notice a thorny resistance to changing our point of view because it can be so satisfying to be right. Or we play the victim by fingering our wounds and showing off our scars as proof of how badly we've been treated. Practicing this fourth attitude doesn't mean we forego healthy discrimination in our relationships or that we stay in abusive or unhealthy partnerships. It just means that we don't have to hold on to the story and harbor ill will toward another. By expounding on the behavior of others, we fortify our ill will and encase ourselves in bitterness. As one friend related, harboring resentment is like drinking poison and waiting for the other person to die.[2]

The fourth *brahmavihara* looks at how we inflict suffering on ourselves and how we manufacture our own torment by failing to detach ourselves from things that ultimately we cannot change in another.

When an extended member of my family failed to acknowledge my brother's death in any way, either by note, phone call, or visit, I began to harbor a resentment that grew into full-blown hatred. I justified my daydreams of revenge by recalling the ways in which I had supported this person through the loss of three of her own family members. It was inconceivable to me how someone living only ten minutes from my home, knowing my brother had died an excruciating death from cancer, could act as if nothing had happened. I concluded that her behavior was unconscionable and therefore unforgivable. It was not hard to find support for this point of view as I bandied my story of mistreatment to all who would listen. Daydreaming one afternoon, I imagined what I might do if I saw her walking on the street and was alarmed to find myself steering my imaginary car onto the sidewalk and running her over. "What was that bump?" I laughed, continuing on my merry way. When twelve months later these violent reveries persisted, I decided it was time to act. Any attempt in meditation to harbor loving thoughts toward her were thwarted by an avalanche of anger and further stories about all the other things she had done. When would I let go of these feelings? Who was suffering here?

Patanjali did not go as far as Christ in advising us to love our enemies: he offered a more realistic solution. At the very least, he advised, develop tolerance toward others. Maybe we're not capable or ready to love these people, but developing detachment so that we're not spinning our wheels can be a very high practice. And we can be creative in finding that tolerance. I decided that it seemed easiest to imagine forgiving my relative once she was dead, so for many weeks I imagined sitting by her coffin and trying to feel empathy for her. I tried to imagine what had happened in her own life to make her so hardened and callous. I thought about her loneliness and how she had no real friends, since she was unable to establish any intimacy with others. I wondered about how acknowledging my grief might have been frightening for her, perhaps opening the floodgates of all her own unexpressed grief. I did these practices, not for her, but to alleviate my own suffering. These meditations did not result in liking her any more than I had before, but my active participation with my anger diminished, until one day I picked up the phone and decided to wish her a happy new year. I did not have the courage to visit her. But somehow hearing her small human voice over the phone broke the last vestiges of my resentment. Nothing had changed in her behavior, and she had not acknowledged my brother's death. But my own changed way of seeing left me with a deep sense of relief. As I dropped the heavy burden of resentment, I felt a new energy and lightness.

The fourth *brahmavihara* is based on the understanding that whatever we refuse in another, we essentially refuse within ourselves. That which we fear, despise, and hate in another, we fear, despise, and hate within ourselves. I have no doubt that each of us, given unfortunate circumstances, has the ability to become a murderer, an abuser, or a fraud. When we can reclaim the dimensions of ourselves that are the necessary polarities of love, compassion, and kindness, we can better accept these traits in others. This doesn't mean we condone them or allow their expression, it simply means that we honestly recognize these potentials in ourselves. Then we are less likely to react to the behavior of others.

Like the *yamas* and *niyamas,* the ethical and moral practices that create the conditions for living a sane and soulful life, practicing the *brahmavihara* fosters the conditions for the mind to become tranquil. Patanjali gives us many other useful practices, but he wisely realized that none of the other practices was likely to work very well if our minds were caught up in the anger, fear, or defensiveness born out of living a "me" and "thee" existence. No matter how wonderful our Yoga postures look or how long we can sit in meditation, these attainments are erased when we cut someone off in traffic or steal the Yoga mat as we're leaving class. If the breeding ground of all the other causes of suffering is "not-seeing" (*avidha*) our fundamental sameness, what better solution than to reverse this tendency by practicing friendliness, loving-kindness, and detachment born of acceptance?

Patanjali gives us a starting point and, as we shall see, a host of methods and approaches to try on for size, but he leaves one rather important detail up to us. And this, ironically, is the most important detail of all. How do we find the volition to practice? We turn now to the question of how to transform motive into motivation and aspiration into attainment.

Chapter 7

The Freedom of Discipline

Until one is committed, there is hesitancy, the chance to draw back, always ineffectiveness concerning all acts of initiative and creation. There is one elementary truth the ignorance of which kills countless ideas and splendid plans: that the moment one definitely commits oneself, then providence moves too. All sorts of things occur to help one that would never otherwise have occurred. A whole stream of events issues from the decision, raising in one's favor all manner of unforeseen incidents and meetings and material assistance which no man could have dreamed would have come his way. Whatever you can do or dream you can, begin it. Boldness has genius, power and magic in it. Begin it now.

Goethe

Discipline is a decidedly unpopular notion these days, associated as it is with self-coercion and denial of pleasure. Far from the punitive and constricting connotations of the word as it is used today, the Latin origin of the word discipline, *disciplina*, means "to impart knowledge" and "to enlighten." This gives us a very different insight into the purpose of discipline. Rather than constraining, discipline is any practice that *contains* our thoughts, energy, and actions so that we can use ourselves in a potent way. Just as a bucket riddled with holes cannot carry water from one place to another, lack of containment of our physical, psychological, and psychic energies sabotages our best intentions.

Most of us think that to discipline our lives would mean to dampen all the good fun we are having. We may see discipline on one side of the ledger as limiting our choices and imagine the credit side as full of marvelous and spontaneous possibilities. We might notice that whenever we try to give a clear structure and shape to our actions, a subtle (and sometimes not-so-subtle) inner conflict pulls us almost instantly in a contradictory direction. What pulls us in this opposing direction is actually a healthy longing for the *feeling* of freedom. This longing is a vital and necessary component of any spiritual quest. We may so want this feeling of lightness and joy in our lives that we rush headlong and grab for whatever and whoever will provide us with some semblance of this feeling. Yet this ersatz freedom is like drinking salty water—the more we drink, the more we feel thirsty. When we channel our energy, we start to use this same longing and desire in a way that can bring deep satisfaction.

An important part of learning to channel our energies is *increasing our tolerance for staying in the pause between desire and satisfaction.* This is a very important point. For some of us, even a momentary delay in quenching our longing can cause a feeling of inner panic. Just as a person trying to quit smoking may struggle to overcome the urge to smoke, when we contain desire we begin to understand what it is that we really crave and how we might put an end to that craving. An essential element of increasing our skillfulness in this domain is learning to be in the pause between a feeling and a reaction.

What happens in the pause between the longing for a feeling of freedom and how we respond to that longing is worth considering further because it is in this pause that we make a choice. For instance, we may come home from work, and the moment we find the house empty we feel a twinge of loneliness. We might feel a physical lassitude or mental fatigue from the demands of our workday. Or we might actually feel a pleasant silence within ourselves. Let us imagine that something in us wants comfort or a lightening of spirit. This is a potent moment that many of us experience daily, if not hourly—the moment of feeling a longing for happiness. If we can get comfortable in being in that pause, however it manifests for us physically, psychologically, and emotionally, we have a better chance of responding to our longing in a way that is not simply a stopgap measure. Maybe we have become accustomed to grabbing for the remote, pouring ourselves a drink, or reaching for the phone. Usually these mechanical strategies simply dull or numb our feeling state. Millions of people worldwide spend a third of their waking lives glued to the TV in a state of physical, mental, and emotional paralysis. What might happen if we had the presence of mind and the wherewithal to really be in that pause and ask what would truly satisfy us? When we contain rather than constantly discharge our feeling state, we allow ourselves to feel completely. In feeling completely, we reexperience our aliveness and the source of that aliveness. When we cultivate the discipline to pause, it becomes possible for us to make a choice that is outside our normal habit pattern. And it is in breaking through these entrained patterns that we can begin to experience a more liberated state of being. Gradually we become the freedom that we previously longed for.

According to tantric teaching (the esoteric practice of activating one's innate spiritual energy), mind and *prana* (the life force behind all movement) manifest as two aspects of unity. Mind is that which is aware, *prana* the active energy that gives support to the awareness. When we learn to master the mind, we automatically master the movement of *prana*, and vice versa. The aim of any system of meditation or spiritual attunement is to master this movement of awareness. What we discipline, then, is this movement of awareness, training ourselves to stay with rather than run from all that we experience. When we choose to stay with our practice despite the inevitable highs and lows in our lives, we are actively choosing to focus our awareness on that part of us that is unchanging. With each practice session, we start to identify with this steady part of ourselves. When we're feeling sad, we practice anyway. When we're happy and excited, we practice anyway. When we're in the depths of grief, we practice anyway. When we have a thousand things to do, we practice anyway. We do not practice to rid ourselves of these feelings or to suppress them. Neither do we practice out of stoic denial. When we practice through thick and thin, happy and unhappy times, we are saying, "Sadness is moving through me, but sadness is not who I am; excitement is moving through me, but excitement is not who I am; grief is moving through me, but grief is not only who I am." When we practice anyway, we make room to fully experience all our feelings while at the same time not allowing those feelings to paralyze or solidify into our identity.

This paying attention to the ground of the mind is like observing the sky rather than the things in it. We may notice a bird flying through the sky, but certainly the sky does not become smudged from this movement. Today it is rainy, but somehow the sky does not become wet. Tomorrow it is sunny, but the sky doesn't ignite into flames. The next day there is an exciting show of thunder and lightning, yet no one rushes around trying to repair the sky. In the same way, when we have the discipline to stay with our practice, we insist on remaining identified with our own neutral witness, the part of us that stays the same regardless of the passing show.

Yoga tells us that our biggest obstacle in perceiving reality as it is is our habit of identifying with and participating in the stuff that fills our mind. And what is this mind-stuff? Latent impressions are left in our minds from past experiences in the form of memories, which tend to dictate our way of seeing things in the present and thus further determine the shape of our future. As if our minds are not already filled to the brim with these past impressions, we further complicate our mind state by making things up, filling the mind with fantasies and fears about things that haven't yet happened. The habit of participating in all of this tomfoolery itself forms more latent impressions, which strengthens our conviction that this is who we are. It is as if we have become so used to dressing in masquerade that we start to see ourselves as our fantasy character.

When we establish a habit of shifting this identification so that we participate with the background of thought, the silent ground of consciousness, this too forms an impression. Just as the impressions left by the constant stream of thoughts and sensations tend to propel more of the same, the impressions left through participation with the silent substrate of consciousness generates a flow of itself. Silence begins to flow through us as our fundamental state of being. This is as it has always been. Nothing new has been created; we simply have cleared a pathway through which this silence can flow and regenerate itself. This new impression, like the sky, is itself impressionless. It does not offer itself as a ground for collecting new material. What began as outer-imposed discipline (that is, what we have to do to shift the mind's focus) becomes an inner discipline that generates itself. This Self-generative process is always fresh and original, giving us the freedom to be and act authentically.

There is a wonderful story about Milarepa, the eleventh-century Buddhist poet, saint, and yogi who reached enlightenment in his lifetime. This was rather an extraordinary accomplishment given that at various times in his life Milarepa was a scoundrel: a murderer, a thief, a liar, a suicidal depressive—in essence, someone most of us could relate to. Yet Milarepa managed to harness his energy with such masterful awareness that he became one of Tibet's most cherished teachers. A young man who had the good fortune to meet Milarepa was so moved by his accomplishments that he offered his most valued possession, his beautiful horse. The young man said to Milarepa:

> To a man of the world, a good horse is his pride.
> I give you this fine horse as an offering,
> Praying that you may keep me from the hell
> Into which I else would fall.

To which Milarepa replied:

> A horse of Prana-Mind have I;
> I adorn him with the silk scarf of Dhyana.
> His skin is the magic Ensuing Dhyana Stage,
> His saddle, illuminating Self-Awareness.
> My spurs are the Three Visualizations,
> His crupper the secret teaching of the Two Gates.

His head stall is the Prana of Vital-force,
His forelock curl is Three-pointed Time.
Tranquility within is his adornment,
Bodily movement is his rein,
And ever-flowing inspiration is his bridle.
He gallops wildly along the Spine's Central Path.
He is a yogi's horse, this steed of mine.
By riding him, one escapes Samsara's mud.
By following him, one reaches the safe land of Bodhi.[1]

Notice that the end result of Milarepa's training is not a quiet carriage horse that hangs its head low but a horse that "gallops wildly" along a central pathway. From this passage we can glean that through the disciplined training of our minds we do not become watered-down versions of our former self or lifeless automatons. Rather, all that is feisty and full of life is now channeled. I have seen this to be true in many long-standing Yoga practitioners: through practice we become truer to who we are—eccentric, idiosyncratic, and "full of our selves."

The untrained habitual mind is often compared to a drunken monkey, but like Milarepa, I like the image of the wild horse better for in this archetype we see the potential for what was once uncontrolled impulsive energy to be channeled into harmonious action. As a horsewoman I have experienced firsthand how disciplined training can transform a potentially lethal animal into a creature of magic that can remove human limitations and give unfathomable joy to her steward. And I have looked on as riders with poorly trained horses spend their mounted hours fighting bucking, balking, and bolting horses. Even as their fingers bleed from the pull of the reins, they will not consider taking the time to retrain their difficult mounts, declaring all the while that they ride for pleasure and not to make it into work. Most will look on in envy at the rider with loose reins and relaxed horse, convinced that this accomplishment is sheer luck or that the rider simply "got a good horse." It is like the old adage: The harder I work, the luckier I get. In the same way, I have overheard Yoga students admire the accomplished demonstration of a Yoga *asana*, or posture, as if it had come floating down a stream in a basket and wonder how they too could get so lucky. If we look at the admirable traits and accomplishments of others, we almost always find a commitment to disciplined practice. It is only when we are willing to be honest with ourselves and give up the artifice that we're having a good time that we can give ourselves wholeheartedly to the task at hand. This is the beginning of getting our energy to work for us rather than against us.

Regardless of the specific form of meditation we choose or the specific style or tradition of Yoga we practice, we can begin to channel our energy by asking the question "Are my choices supporting what is deeply satisfying in my life?" And are my choices leading to long-term freedom or short-lived pleasure? If we went through an average day asking these questions, our day might look quite different. These kinds of questions lead us to evaluate what is important to us and to choose to what purpose we will devote our time and energy. When we're tempted to press the snooze alarm button, we can ask whether thirty minutes' more sleep will bring us the same results as thirty minutes of practice. If we don't have the energy for practice, why not? Do we awaken feeling tired because we overate or overimbibed the night before, or do we chronically overwork so that we feel depleted and irritable all the time? Can we take responsibility for the untold ways we cop out and sabotage ourselves? When students of Baba Hari Dass (the longtime silent sadhu and spiritual leader of Mount Madonna Center in California) asked him how they could get out of bed early enough to practice, he responded by writing on his chalkboard, "Get up at 5 A.M. every day no matter what, and after a while you will go to bed at 10!"

When we sidestep our practice, what are we escaping from? When we can't make time to practice, what are we avoiding? Usually we are escaping from all the little demons that have set up shop in our minds and hearts who are currently having a reckless fiesta party and the

drinks are on us. We may also be escaping from a feeling we find uncomfortable or from the very questions that might lead us to reassess
our lives. Often these feelings have to do with a terrible sense of
meaninglessness and emptiness that we try to fill or cover up. Any
evasion will do as long as it serves to deflect and delay experiencing
the source of our unease. Or we have a deeply ingrained unconscious
fear of failure, and taking the risk to make a go of anything that really
matters to us puts us smack-dab in the middle of our fear.

So when we insist on getting up early in the morning, when we insist on staying with our meditation for the time we agreed, and when
we insist on practicing *asanas* each day, we make space to visit these
questions. And we can be assured that when we begin to insist on this
new game plan, the executive ego will predictably balk. It is too cold,
too hot, too late, too early, too noisy, or, heaven forbid, it is too quiet.
Or we are too stiff, too hungry, too tired, too nervous, too busy, too
bored, too distracted, or too upset to practice. When we hear our
executive ego whispering these endless excuses and evasions, we can
make note of the excuse and do our practice anyway. We can develop
a sense of humor when we hear ourselves come up with the wildest
evasions, and then do our practice anyway. This is how we begin to
rein in the mind. As we learn to rein in the mind and rein in our actions, we gain control over our lives once again.

It would be unbalanced to say that practice is simply about facing
our demons or facing what is unpleasant, unfinished, or unresolved in
our lives. As the mind becomes centered in its own stillness, we rediscover the intrinsic loveliness of the mind and how wonderful it is to
go through the day with the support of such a centered mind. As the
body becomes strong, flexible, and relaxed, we rediscover the joy of
physical vitality and how wonderful it is to be able to do all the things
we enjoy without restriction. Through ever increasing skillfulness, we
become more adaptable and improvisational in response to life's demands. But it is not just the positive aftereffects of the practice that
can keep us motivated, it is the deep satisfaction and solace within the
practice itself. And it is the gradual cessation of conflict as we learn

to inhabit the pause between desire and satisfaction and discover that therein lies fullness. As we become that which we seek, there is no one and no thing left to discipline.

Why then can it be so hard to devote ourselves to sustained practice? Resistance to practice occurs when we have not yet formed a clear intention. Until we form a clear intention, we cannot rally our energy and align it with our goal. We have to know what it is that we really want. We may say we're practicing Yoga because we want to lose weight or become flexible or fit. But until we understand that what we really want is to feel truly alive, there will always be a contrary movement that pulls us in a negative direction. Once we find the core of our intention, this intention acts like a laser to cut through the endless excuses and evasions. We stop having a devil on one shoulder and an angel on the other, battling it out in a tit-for-tat competition. Instead, we align ourselves from the center of our intention, and the friction of opposing forces ceases to obstruct our momentum.

When we avoid practice we often are also failing to distinguish between stimulation and agitation. We may mistakenly interpret agitation as stimulation, and, further, we may interpret peacefulness as dullness. Once a friend sympathetically shared how hard it must be for me to live in the country, where "nothing ever happens." I assured her that every day my garden was a theater of sensual drama: colors changing, seasons shifting, the sounds of birds and wildlife. I countered by asking her how stimulating she found her two-hour commute to work. It is understandable that we may come to feel threatened by the cusp of peacefulness, given the relentless way in which most of us are bombarded with stimuli throughout the course of a normal day. We may find the hubbub perversely reassuring, as if all this commotion were some evidence of a meaningful life. We may unconsciously view disciplined practice or ordering our lives as staid compared to the seemingly glittering attraction of going out to the movies or to the shopping mall, but how often do we return from such sojourns feeling empty-hearted?

A participant once arrived at an intensive Yoga retreat declaring that her whole life was in a chaotic mess. Her body felt battered by poor diet and lack of exercise, and the stress of her high-powered job had left her so filled with anxiety that she needed sleeping pills to get to sleep and tranquilizers to function during the day. On the one day of the retreat in which participants had an opportunity to practice silence, she chose instead to leave the retreat site to wine and dine at a local hot spot with a few other talkative companions. Curiously, after a few days on the retreat she proclaimed, "I long to corrupt you." I wondered whether the measured lifestyle of the retreat setting translated in her mind into a kind of death and it was this interpretation that made it so hard for her to lead a more balanced life.

Whether our discipline grants us greater freedom or not depends on what drives us to practice. Are we driven by fear or by joy? Are we driven by a terror of the magnitude of life and an attempt to make our lives small enough that we feel safe? Or are we driven by a longing to become big enough and strong enough to endure the larger life that is possible for us? If we use our practice to shield ourselves from the world or to obsessively control and suppress our real thoughts and feelings, no amount of practice will bring about the happiness we desire. When our practice is driven by a need to make our entire life predictable and secure, the results will be psychologically and spiritually stifling.

Years ago I invited a very respected teacher to come and share his knowledge with my students. This teacher was revered for his strict practice regimen—indeed, he had a little book detailing exactly what he was going to do every day of the week. Although the technical information he had to impart was of value, it soon became apparent that his foremost concern was in adhering to his own practice schedule. Such was his obsession that one afternoon he got up while the class was still in relaxation pose, got dressed, and left—all so he could keep to his exacting routine. His instructions were almost unanimously negative: offering a litany of all the things the students needed to correct without offering the kind of praise that encourages the effort necessary to make changes. At the end of the intensive, when it is traditional for the teacher to thank the students and for the students to have a chance to show their appreciation, he dashed out the door without so much as a good-bye. The students, who had given him their fullest attention for three days, were disheartened. Perhaps the questions that this incident provoked were as valuable as the intensive itself.

After this experience, I began to wonder about my own perfectionist tendencies and harsh standards. Any practice can be used as a shield to protect us from life. Discipline can be just as effective as sloth in helping us escape from reality: we can schedule, control, and otherwise fill up our day with so many plans that there is not even the smallest crack for an outside influence to seep in. If we find that any variation in our routine evokes a sense of insecurity, then we may be using discipline to cordon ourselves off from the greater challenge of securing our spiritual practice in the ground of everyday life. Achieving a dynamic balance between aspiration and actuality can be our gauge for knowing whether or not our discipline is setting us free.

Chapter 8

Embodied Awareness

So what is to be done?
I'm suggesting a return to a primordial language.
One that exists as the deepest knowledge and expression that humanity
*   knows.*
It predates spoken language, it has its roots in the emergence of awe.
It is present in everyone, as an elemental music and reflection of
*   molecular and stellar movement.*
It is a genetic design built into leaf patterns and the bobbing of sea
*   horses.*
It is eminently present to children, we have educated it out of them.
But it is the story of our place in the universe and we must begin to
*   tell that story again.*
What we are losing is our ability to speak to the whole.
The songs of celebration, the poetry of praise.

                    Author unknown

When we live in exile from the sensate reality of the body, we live in
exile from the source of our aliveness. The only place that we can reconnect with this aliveness is in the body. Of course we all have bodies, yet few of us truly inhabit our bodies. We may live a short
distance from the body divorced from our feelings, sensations, intuitions, and instincts. The body may seem like a foreign land that we
have read about but never personally visited. And just as we may come
to know a foreign land through the stories we've heard and the pictures we've seen, the actual reality of the place can never be known
until we have walked, eaten, smelled, touched, and been there ourselves. When we begin to live in the body again, we take up citizen-

ship in our personal residence. In this way we come home to the body.

When we are not at home in our body, we divest ourselves of our somatic reality. Because the body is the only place where we can have access to our feelings and thoughts, ignoring our body affords us some distance from the content of our inner world. We may unconsciously believe that leaving the body is one way of leaving all those onerous feelings and thoughts behind. Unfortunately, in disassociating from what may be painful, we also disassociate from what may be pleasurable. Even if we do pay attention to our bodies, this attention may be steeped in negativity. As one student admitted, "The only two parts of my body I like are my nose and my ankles." Or we may ignore or deflect the feelings that arise from our body. All of these strategies not only distance us from our most immediate reality, our physical body, they distance us from life itself. When we begin to live in the body again, we discover that we have an internal environment that is as rich as that of any country and in a constant state of flux and change.

We would do well to ask why so many of us drop our bodies long before our mortal end. When the body is viewed as an apparatus for carrying the head around, we leave ourselves prone to the tyranny of our intellect and the justification and defense of the rational mind. This may give us a nifty sense of control over our lives. While the rational mind is a necessary instrument for discriminative awareness, it is not the only means by which we come to know something. We also come to know through the feeling in our gut, the hair that rises on our neck, or a "sense" that tells us to get out now. The rational mind houses our ego, and a well-developed ego gives us a healthy sense of our own worthiness and is of itself a good thing to have. The rational mind gives our thoughts some grounding, which is also a good thing.

Yet the rational mind also houses our executive ego, which sees itself as the protector of our "I." This executive ego does not take lightly to anyone or anything interfering with its dictates. This part of the ego manifests largely as puffed-up self-importance and spends a great deal of its time defending its "self." As the representative of the executive ego, the rational mind has the advantage of being highly trained, frequently exercised (and obeyed), and, not so incidentally, heavily invested in perpetuating its own dominant position in the chain of command.

By the time most of us have reached early adulthood, our executive ego has had a doctorate education while our bodily instincts may still be in kindergarten. We may have become accustomed to ignoring or overriding our inner instincts, mainly because they do not tally with the grand plan of our executive ego. Our mind may tell us that it's a good idea to stay at our job for exactly three more years, but our body may have other thoughts on the matter. The executive ego tells us to plow through our fatigue even if it's the first day of a difficult period, while the body cries out for an afternoon nap. We may become such experts at living outside the reach of our bodily instincts that we start to navigate our lives purely from our rational minds, leaving behind our gut instincts and our heartfelt desires. Our inner wisdom, which is guided by the body, does not take lightly to this dismissal. Navigating our lives with only one instrument of perception is like setting out on a journey across the ocean with a compass while ignoring the movement of the wind, water, and stars. In the Katha Upanishad we're told that there is a physical location to this inner wisdom:

That through which one enjoys form,
Taste, smell, sound,
Touch, and sexual union is the Self.
Can there be anything not known to That
who is the One in all?
    Katha Upanishad 2.3[1]

Unlike many spiritual and religious traditions, which further disenfranchise us from the support of our embodied self, Yoga stands apart as a tradition that has always recognized the importance of the body and mind living in harmonious relationship to each other. Yogis recognized that the physical manifestation of the body was but a form animated by something greater than itself. The same force that moves the tides, opens a flower, or creates lightning in a storm animates our bodies. This life force moves the breath, the fluids, and the current flowing through our nerves as well as the inner workings of each and every cell. This animating principle is the force behind all the organs of perception: hearing, touch, taste, smell, and sight. Although not itself a solid substance, this life force infuses the body and manifests as the light shining from our eyes, the glow of the skin, and the timbre of the voice. As this force moves through the body, it influences the shape and form of our structure, creating our posture, the rhythm of our walk, and the character of our faces. Everything that has ever happened to us—our birth, the fall from a tree at the age of six, our thoughts and feelings, what we eat, the climate in which we live—is inscribed upon our body, creating a living archaeological record. When we develop an awareness of the interior movement that permeates the body, we gain access to the movement of our minds. Yoga is a means of reviving our connection to this natural wisdom.

When we practice the *asanas*, or Yoga postures, we begin to reunite ourselves once again with the contents of consciousness. Through rejoining the body, we learn to become internally literate once again. The physical literacy that Yoga offers us goes far beyond that recognized by Western science. Such was the uncompromising belief of ancient yogis that every part of the body could become conscious, was indeed consciousness itself, that they mapped an inner geography of the body that reflected the force behind form. They were interested not just in the function of the organs and tissues but also in the way in which the elements of nature—earth *(prithvi)*, water *(ap)*, fire *(tejas)*, air *(vayu)*, and space *(akash)*—interacted with one another, and how a balance or imbalance of these elements created health or disease. Just as the laws and regulations that govern the orderly working of a city are invisible yet nonetheless determine the direction, shape, and form of all action, the yogis were interested in discovering the underlying laws of nature. In doing so they recognized different layers, or *koshas*, to the body—interpenetrating frequencies from the gross flesh to the most subtle energetic infrastructures. They also recognized that the *prana*, or life force infusing the body, moved in particular directions and that the subtle control of this life force could shape the movement of consciousness. Thus, becoming aware of the physical body was not distinguished from awareness of consciousness itself.

In the West we have come to view the body as an object, to exercise "it" as a separate entity from ourselves, and to command and control the body. This extract from *The Human Body*, a book designed to educate children, sums it up:

> You can think of your body as a space capsule with your head as the command module and your trunk as the service module. Your head contains your brain, the computer which guides and controls the human space mission. . . . The brain also has control centers which govern the machinery in the service module. They automatically regulate the rate and rhythm of your heart and your breathing and tell you when to drink and when to eat. As you can see, the computer in your head controls your life.[2]

When the body becomes an "it," we become someone doing something to somebody—always in a state of disassociation. Further, our definition of physical fitness has primarily focused on the superficial appearance of the body. So obsessed are we with this reductionistic view of the body that we have videos whose sole purpose is to produce "buns of steel" or "abs to die for" and books promising a "hard body." This obsessive attention to what can be seen on the exterior prevents us from developing the kind of interior awareness that gives us access to our deepest insights. Further, the physical armoring of the body so common in our models of fitness causes a numbing of subtler sensation and feeling and, not so coincidentally, dampens any possible awareness we might cultivate of deeper body systems.

Nowhere in the entire literature of Yoga do we see this preoccupation with the outer wrappings of the body. Rather, the fitness of the gross, or *annamaya kosha,* layer of the body is inferred from the inner health of the subtle body.

> Health, a light body, freedom from craving,
> A glowing skin, sonorous voice, fragrance
> Of body: these signs indicate progress
> In the practice of meditation.
> > Shvetashvatara Upanishad 2.12[3]

In the Yoga-Sutra we are told that bodily perfection manifests as beauty, grace, a diamondlike glow, and supreme strength (3.46).

If we imagine the body as a community, with each body system and each layer a representative of consciousness, our Western expression of the body is limited almost entirely to the loudmouth of the body representatives, the musculoskeletal system, while the other internal systems such as the organs, fluids, and glands remain veritable wallflowers within our awareness. Since the musculoskeletal system is energized by the sympathetic nervous system (the part of the central nervous system responsible for fright, fight, flight, or a fake-it response), when we are in our muscle mind we tend to operate from the high notes of our nervous system. Our sympathetic nervous system is primarily engaged with sensing what is "out there" and in protecting us from danger. Primarily existing in and expressing ourselves from this exterior level keeps our attention chronically focused outward. Without the base support of our parasympathetic nervous system, which governs respiration, relaxation, and functions such as digestion, our somatic reality can become ungrounded. For this reason, the *asanas,* or Yoga postures, were traditionally practiced very slowly, with each movement synchronized to the breath, in order to balance the nervous system and open a perceptual gateway to the parasympathetic nervous system. This makes us available to our feeling function.

When we practice *asanas* from an interior perspective, we bring our minds back into the body. Instead of directing the body as a separate entity, we relocate our minds within our body and begin to listen to the nonverbal, nonmental information contained within the soma. As we give our full attention to every breath, movement, and the subtlest of sensations, the body becomes mindful, and the mind becomes embodied. In so doing, we directly experience the body as an opaque form of consciousness, and we start to see the intimate relationship between the contents of what we think, feel, and imagine and our physical reality. In this reconciliation between body and mind we begin to experience a unitive rather than divisive state. This is what distinguishes the authentic practice of hatha Yoga from mere stretching. If we read a book or watch TV while our body marches on the treadmill, we actually create a form of mental and physical retardation and reinforce our disconnection from our body wisdom.

Since our Western cultural inheritance precludes a whole relationship to the body, it is not at all surprising that hatha yoga here has often been reinvented as a sophisticated form of calisthenics whose sole purpose is to make the body beautiful and to increase longevity. These things hatha yoga does well, but such goals are not the primary goal of yoga practice, and when we practice in a way that causes this unhealthy identification with the body, we are merely doing exercises with Sanskrit names. The practice becomes bent to accommodate the perception of the body as an "it" rather than requiring us to bend our minds and stretch beyond our objectified perceptual leanings. When our primary imperative shifts from attaining a form to developing an intimate connection with the life force moving through that form, we are reclaiming the *only* part of the practice that ultimately can have any relevance for us—finding out who we really are. And for this purpose hatha yoga is an exceptional system for becoming aware not only of the body but also of the life force that animates it and us.

The limitless nature of consciousness is mirrored in the *asana* repertoire itself. A testament to the vast creativity of our yogic forebears, the repertoire is drawn from nature, with each posture representing some aspect or expression of creation. We practice being the expression of trees, insects, birds, mammals, children, sages, gods, and mountains. Every *asana* that has come down to us today began with an authentic inner impulse that was felt and experienced by someone at some time and then recorded so that it might be shared. Literally translated as "comfortable seat," the word *asana* means to relax into the consciousness of life as it manifests through the expression of each posture.

When we practice *asanas* we try to rediscover the origin of each movement and thus the original meaning of each gesture. This discovery cannot be made by simply mimicking another person or mechanically reproducing the postures. For the *asanas* to transform us, we enter the total feeling state of that form. By becoming a fish, bird, tree, or mountain, we reinvoke our connectedness with all creation at each stage of evolution.

The process of practicing *asanas* can be codified into a number of distinct stages that we progressively cycle through. The stages build in successive layers, with each stage providing a platform for the support of the next.

FEELING WHAT IS

When we enter an *asana* we start by feeling what is. We observe the mind-body entity from a neutral viewpoint, resting our attention like dust settling on a table, lightly and without pressure. When we observe from this neutral vantage point, the process of perception has no ideal and no agendas. We simply feel how we are and offer ourselves complete acceptance for whatever we are bringing to the mat. When we can bring an accepting presence to our observations we begin the process of befriending ourselves. This is a crucial first step, for without this neutral witness we cannot possibly know how we actually are, and thus we cannot know where to begin or how to skillfully work with ourselves in the practice. If we do not extend this goodwill toward ourselves our practice will always be a time of frustration and disappointment. Because of the neutrality of the witness, observation has the possibility of extending beyond our habitual thought patterns. As we develop choiceless awareness we begin to see things not as we imagine they should be but as they really are.

FEELING WHERE WE ARE STUCK

When we first enter a posture we are met by our ability or inability to take on this new form. We feel all the places where we hold tension. These areas of accumulated tension represent the repetition of our ideation process, that is, our thoughts, fears, tensions, and anxieties coalescing into distinct patterns of tension and form our unique individual posture or attitude to life. As we think, so we become. We also encounter the history of the body in the form of traumas from birth, injuries, illness, and emotional disruption from the past and present, and we open to the possibility that we can move beyond these limitations. So the first experience we have when we practice an *asana* is awareness of the places that do not yet yield beyond the perimeters of our current expression. This is often a discomforting moment. Our idea about how pleasant it will be to take a Yoga class often meets reality the very first time we bend forward and feel the excruciating pull of our hamstring muscles. If this were all that happened, there would be a very high attrition rate indeed, but fortunately we have the opportunity to go a step further by entering into a dialogue with this tension.

JOINING WITH THE BREATH

We begin to join our awareness with the breath and to use the breath to "palpate" and feel places of tension. As we breathe we start to realize that there are three phases to each breath—arising, dissolving, and pausing. As we take in the symphony of sensation, we learn to synchronize our practice so that we expand with the incoming breath, relax effort on the outgoing breath, and pause in the silence between these two phases. As we become adept at uniting our breath, body, and mind into one action, we become intimate with the natural rhythm of life as it arises out of stillness, manifests into form, and then dissolves back into stillness. We start to become comfortable with the fact that everything is changing and in flux and that we can ride this fluctuation skillfully. We also begin to understand that as sensations, thoughts, and feelings pass through us, they need not solidify. They need not bunch up inside us as knots of tension. We can be a person who occasionally feels tension rather than a tense person. That is, all of these passing sensations need not concretize and fuse our identity. As we become more accomplished, the body consciousness becomes more malleable, able to adapt and assume whatever expression most skillfully serves the moment.

REFINING OUR RELATIONSHIP WITH THE LIFE FORCE

As we become more adept, we refine our position in each posture so that *prana*, or life force, moves through us clearly and with ease. To do this we must clarify our relationship to the ground, to gravity, and to space and also clarify the harmonious relationship between each part of the body to the whole. This involves finding a dynamic tension whereby we become effective conduits for the animating movement of *prana*. We are quite literally in the process of realigning ourselves with the rhythm of the universe. Having fallen out of sync with this primordial rhythm, we try to reestablish a harmony between ourselves and the world. This harmony is expressed when we can sit with elegance, stand erect, walk with grace, and lie down with ease.

This reanimation of the body cannot happen merely through putting the body in a position. Finding our natural rhythm happens through inquiry that is marked by curiosity, innocence, and playfulness. When we bring these three qualities to our inquiry, we start to get more and more comfortable with not knowing. The executive ego begins to relax, and our external commands drop away so we can become receptive to the information coming through the wisdom body.

We know instinctively how to align our bodies—how to open up our blocks and holding places. A teacher can help us tap into this awareness, but ultimately finding our inner alignment is just that: an inside job. If we are receptive, the body will suggest to us subtle shifts of position that can bring about a better alignment. The key here is that we have to trust our inner instincts and stop overriding them with our intellect. Instead of directing the movement from the ambition of the habitual mind (invested as it so often is in quantity rather than quality, goal rather than process), we direct the movement through sensing and feeling and moment-to-moment deduction. Through this inner guidance, we learn to wait for opening moments when the body says *yes* and allows us to go farther into a movement. We also learn to pause respectfully at the edge of our resistance and to listen to the body's *no*. Working in this way, we open up new pathways without injuring ourselves, and because the body has ushered us into this new opening, it will undoubtedly be a change that we can integrate into our whole being.

MOVING INTO STILLNESS

As our work with *asanas* becomes yet more refined, we redirect our awareness to the stillness that is in between, inside, and throughout all movement. This awareness is most readily available when we sit in meditation, hold a posture, or become conscious of the still pause between two breaths. In later stages of practice our awareness of this stillness becomes omnipresent. This experience of stillness within the movement can happen anytime we become completely merged with the movement itself. This is not an experience we can make happen but one that happens through sustained practice and through grace. Eventually, we are not only aware of stillness, we *are* stillness.

If practiced with a conscious awareness of the purpose of Yoga, which is to realize a unitive state, concentrated *asana* practice, the third limb of Ashtanga Yoga, will naturally involve each of the other seven limbs of practice, especially the ten ethical precepts of the *yamas* and *niyamas* (the first two limbs). Through the practice of *asanas* we can learn to be accepting of our limitations *(ahimsa)*, truthful in our commitment to do our best *(satya)*, and content regardless of the outcome *(santosha)*. We can bring our burning enthusiasm and curiosity *(tapas)* to the practice and look deeply at our reactions and responses to difficulty or ease *(swadhyaya)* and ultimately surrender up our practice to something greater than ourselves *(ishvarapranidhana)*. When we find our right relationship to the ground, gravity, and space, the breath is experienced as a whole-body phenomenon. When this happens we begin to feel ourselves as conduits for the life force and there is energetic continuity throughout our bodies *(pranayama, the fourth limb of Yoga)*. As we delve deeper, the practice of *asana* involves consciously moving into stillness *(pratyahara, the fifth limb)*, focusing our attention on one thing at a time *(dharana, the sixth limb)*, and sustaining this awareness regardless of what is going on around us *(dhyana, the seventh limb)*. When a posture has been perfected, an absolute balance is struck between effort and noneffort, the result of which is a neutralization of all sensation. When this happens the mind returns to original silence *(samadhi, the eighth limb)*. There is no one left to do the pose, only the pose itself moving through us.

Coming home to the body through *asana* practice can be a joyous reunion. For many it will feel like seeing a dear friend after many years of absence. For others it will be a reunion fraught with emotion. As the discursive mind moves into the shadows of consciousness, the body is allowed to speak its mind. When we allow ourselves to experience deep bodily relaxation and the revitalization that accompanies such release, we may experience evocative dreams, whirlwind emotions, and insights that compel action. As a result of these newfound insights we may decide to make changes in our life. Perhaps we decide to change our diet, leave an unsatisfying job, end an unhealthy relationship (or renew our commitment to a good one), or adopt a lifestyle that more clearly reflects our values. We may decide to begin some creative project that has been on the back burner all our lives. In essence, we begin to lead a life that is governed as much by the dictates of the heart and guts as by the rationale of the mind.

We may find that we now have an entirely different navigational system through which to steer our lives. Not only do we have the useful compass of the rational mind, we have the sensate and responsive apparatus of our body to alert us to the subtlest of changes. We start to know what we are feeling and to let our actions be informed by those feelings. We become aware of the first signs of illness and through early intervention have a better chance of preventing full-blown disease. We start to trust that the body has a particular kind of wisdom that we can tune in to if we have the humility to listen. And we start to take into account our bodily wisdom *especially* when it is not congruent with our best-laid plans and to reassess the wisdom of those plans.

While embodied awareness is an integral part of the yogic tradition, yogis have always warned that we should not mistake the map for the territory. We do indeed have a body, but don't make the mistake of thinking that you are *only* your body. From an absolute viewpoint, that which is eternal in us is not the body, but that which is eternal lives *through* the body. If we fail to make this distinction, we will become distraught when our bodies inevitably age or when, through sickness, we are unable to do what was previously possible. There is a beautiful series of affirmations in the Brihadaranyaka Upanishad that teaches us how to make this distinction:

> A wife loves her husband not for his own
> sake, . . . but because the Self lives in him.
> A husband loves his wife not for her own
> sake, . . . but because the Self lives in her.
> Children are loved not for their own sake, but
> because the Self lives in them.
> Wealth is loved not for its own sake,
> but because the Self lives in it.
>
> The universe is loved not for its own sake, but
> because the Self lives in it.

The gods are loved not for their own sake, but
because the Self lives in them.
Creatures are loved not for their own sake, but
because the Self lives in them.
Everything is loved not for its own sake, but
because the Self lives in it.[4]

We might easily add a verse that says:

The body is not loved for its own sake, but
because the Self lives in it.

Yogis were eminently aware of the conundrum of practicing a dispassion toward the body while at the same time recognizing it as the temporary abode of a divine Self. More to the point: Where else but the body *can* we experience consciousness? As Patanjali so clearly lays out in his exposition on the means of attaining a realization of this Self, we have to go through the body; we cannot go around it. And thus, unlike so many traditions that have viewed the body as something to be transcended, the Yoga tradition tells us to make the house of the body a fit place to live.

In recent times the practice of *asana* or hatha yoga has become synonymous with the practice of Yoga. This is unfortunate. The perfection of *asanas* was never meant as the goal of Yoga practice, nor will standing on our head for an hour signal some major achievement on our spiritual path. This misconception is understandable given our obsession with form and our desire to have some kind of concrete evidence of attainment. Traditionally, *asana* practice was only one small sliver of Yoga, yet it was considered a crucial part of practice. Designed to make the body strong yet flexible, alert yet relaxed, the postures gradually fine-tune the body. This fine-tuning calibrates the nervous system so that our senses become extremely discerning. This preparation was considered paramount for beginning the rigors of meditation. It was also recognized that to do such practices as well as to fulfill our duties in the world would take enormous energy, energy that would not be available if we suffered ill health or disease. In this regard the practice of hatha yoga was intended to serve this greater purpose. These practical benefits are of no small consequence. They can make the difference between being able to fulfill our purpose in life or not. Taken out of the larger philosophical context of Yoga as a life practice, however, the *asanas* become nothing more than a glorified stretching regimen.

The point of practicing *asanas* is to become sensitive, attuned, and adaptable. Whether we attain great gymnastic abilities becomes entirely inconsequential in the context of Yoga as a life practice. If we become enamored with the performance of advanced postures and fix our identity on these achievements, we have simply replaced one false identity with another. Many students new to Yoga also make this mistake when choosing a teacher, judging the teacher's qualifications purely through the evidence of his or her ability to do difficult movements. When we realize that what we are advancing toward is not some physical form but an inward recognition of the truth of who we are, then we will not feel ourselves to be failing if we cannot attain difficult postures. *"Advanced" practice is any movement that brings us closer to this recognition of our true self.*

When we keep this larger purpose in mind, the simplest physical practice becomes richly imbued with meaning. We can take great delight in opening the fingers of our hand, in feeling the soles of our feet on the ground, or in the sensation of lightness that comes when we stand erect. Then the body becomes a sacred sanctuary in which that which is worshiped, the worshiper, and the place of worship merge into One.

This oneness is indeed the meaning of the word *Yoga* and is its goal. In following the eight-limb path of Ashtanga Yoga, we have considered the overriding importance of the ten ethical precepts, the *yamas* and *niyamas*, and the way in which our relationships with others accurately reflect our cognition of this unity. We have also looked at the need to discipline our awareness and actions so that we can harness our energies toward this goal. In *asana* practice we embody these understandings, taking them directly into our tissue, bones, and blood so that we experience this unity intimately through our form. The next limb of Ashtanga Yoga, *pranayama*, gives us a practical tool that is always available to us: our breath. Our breath, like our heartbeat, is the most reliable rhythm in our lives. When we become attuned to this constant rhythm, our breath can gradually teach us to come back to the original silence of the mind.

Chapter 9

The Window In

Everything that moves, breathes,
opens and closes
Lives in the Self.

MUNDAKA UPANISHAD 2.1
Translated by Eknath Easwaran

The word *prana* means "constancy in the movement of the life force," and *yama* means "to harness or extend" this force. Thus *pranayama,* the fourth limb of Ashtanga Yoga, is the practice of allowing the breath to move freely; containing and directing the breath toward a specific effect (such as increased vitality); and observing the flow of breath as a lure to bring the mind back to its original source. Although there are thousands of different *pranayama* techniques and breathing practices that involve lengthening, shortening, suspending, and retaining the breath in myriad ways, the foundation of all yogic breathing practices is to establish and maintain a smooth and steady breath rhythm and to apply this skill to everyday living.

Definitions of *pranayama* as breathing exercises or breath control lead us to view the breath as something separate from ourselves. Approached in this way, *pranayama* tends to cause a form of disassociation from rather than a joining with the breath. While a discussion of *pranayama* techniques and practices is beyond the scope of this book, let us look at how an awareness of the breath not only can open us to new levels of vitality but also can help us draw the mind inward. This movement of the mind inward gives us access to our inner wisdom nature. The word *atman,* or inner teacher, is said to derive its etymological roots from the word *an,* "to breathe." This philosophical connection with the word *prana* gives us some sense of the link between opening to our breath and opening to our own natural wisdom.

It begins when we are still in the womb, this expanding, condensing rhythm, threaded together by moments of pause. It is the pulse of the universe, and since our conception we *are* that. While we are in our mother's body, the breath is an interior movement, a process of shimmering cellular respiration. At the moment of birth, when we first breathe into the lungs, we are initiated into the family of things. Suddenly the world is in us and we are in the world. We draw the breath inside the body, for a moment it becomes us, and we exhale a part of what has become us back into the world. While we are young we tend to breathe with the kind of complete freedom and ease that is an expression of our innocence and fearlessness. Yet as we age and lose some of that innocence, rubbing up against life's challenges, we unconsciously shut down, and we achieve this first and foremost by constricting our breath.

For the most part the process of breathing is an unconscious one, which is just as well. None of us would like to stay up all night reminding ourselves to breathe in and out, nor would we have much room for creative thought during the day if we had to do so. But when our breath becomes unconsciously restricted and held, then it can be useful to make this involuntary process conscious. In Yoga practice we do this so we can become aware of our most basic level of aliveness, and as our practice progresses we use a heightened awareness of the breath to train the mind to remain steady with our immediate experience.

When we begin Yoga practice we may notice how often we may hold our breath. Unconsciously restricting the breath indicates that we are out of kilter with life itself. When we hold the breath it is an unconscious attempt to refuse or control our experience. We may get into such a habit of doing this that our breath becomes shallow and we go through the day alternately suffocating and sighing deeply to recover. Or we may be very conscious of our figure, and we chronically contract our belly, causing the breath to move high and tight into the chest. Our breath may become uneven, moving in fits and starts as we alternately open and close to our experience. I often ask my beginning students to make a note for a week of how often they discover themselves holding their breath. Some return a week later flabbergasted. "I hold my breath when I talk, eat, cook, and make the bed." Unless our breathing pattern is caused by a health problem, almost always this holding of the breath represents an unconscious desire for certainty. We hold on to life, and in a sense we hold out on life. And then, of course, life holds out on us.

So even without learning any fancy breathing techniques, just notice how often you close to your most basic connection to life. This will be an invaluable aid in helping you to move back into the stream of life once again. Our next challenge is to allow this ebb and flow to move through us—to gently retrain the breath to become smooth and even once again, and to adapt our breath moment to moment to support our activities. We amplify this process by creating a steady even breath while we are practicing *asanas.* As we come up against the discomfort of tight muscles or challenging positions, we learn to soften and breathe into our tightness or breathe through our difficulty. When an upsetting emotion arises during meditation, we learn to give room for this feeling by allowing our breath to rise and fall. This teaches us that while we cannot control what is going to happen to us, we can control our response. We can choose to open up or to shut down, to soften or to harden.

What we learn on the mat we can then transpose into all our everyday activities. When we get furious and we're about to say something damaging, we pause and steady our breathing. When we're excited, depressed, annoyed, or impatient, we also pause and steady our breathing. When we're in a state of shock or panic, we instinctively know to steady our breathing. This doesn't mean that we necessarily stop feeling shocked or impatient, but through the breath we become aware that there is a neutral background to our feelings and emotions. Consciously making our breath steady at such a time isn't about suppressing our feelings, it is about understanding that every high and every low arises out of and returns back to a potent neutral place. The point is not to control the breath or to control the situation but to use the regular, metronomelike availability of our breath to remind us of the *place inside us that is always steady*. The breath then becomes like a companion that is always reminding us of who we are.

Some years ago I was called to a local hospital by a student whose partner had sustained a severe back injury. She explained as she drove me to the hospital that the doctors had tried four different painkillers, but after almost three hours her husband was still on all fours and unable to move. When we arrived I could see that Len was in a state of panic and that while being on all fours was excruciating, any attempt to lie down caused even more pain. He felt helpless. I gently put my hands on his lower back and asked him to breathe slowly into my hands. The practice of focusing on his breath took his attention away from his growing panic and gradually eased the pain. Soon his back was rising ever so slightly with each inhalation and dropping with each exhalation. I encouraged him to give himself over to the gentle movement of his breath. To his surprise, within minutes he was able to lie on his side and then on his back. Within an hour we had him safely at home. Sadly, it had not occurred to any of the doctors or nurses to help Len in this way. But more important, it had not occurred to Len.

If we use our time on the mat to practice staying with our experience, breathing and opening to each new sensation, whether pleasant or unpleasant, this skill will automatically be there for us when we encounter difficulties in our everyday life. If we haven't developed this skillfulness in the hothouse conditions of practice, then when push comes to shove, like Len, we'll freeze and leave ourselves incapacitated to act skillfully. A friend related how his piano teacher had entered him in a performance without his permission. He showed up for the concert dressed in a flannel shirt and jeans to discover that she had arranged for the two of them to play a duet. Everyone else was dressed in formal attire, and he did not believe himself a capable enough musician to share the stage. Embarrassment turned to anger, which turned to panic. How could she do this to him? Then he re-membered the practice of calming his breath. Gradually the stage fright subsided, and once he calmed down he could see that his teacher was trying to help him. He was not thrilled to be put in such a position, but he went ahead and did the best he could in a tight sit-uation.

Most of us find ourselves in such tight situations on a regular basis. We've had a fight with our partner and we're getting the cold and silent treatment. We get cut off in traffic, or the toilet overflows right before a dinner party, or we're ready to scream because we have three sick kids and one of them has just thrown up on our lap. These are times when we can use our breath to open up and ventilate the sit-uation. We can make a little more room around our experience and in doing so get some perspective.

In Yoga practice we can gain this perspective by using an awareness of our breath to divide our experience into manageable increments. This is how we begin to discipline reality. Or more accurately, we dis-cipline ourselves to choose reality instead of something else that ap-pears more appealing or less painful. While we cannot for one moment stop the world to let us off, we can practice *deliberately simplifying* our experience by just breathing in and out, letting our breath move low and slow. Imagine how difficult it would be to understand a film played at high speed, and you have some sense of the hurricanelike speed with which the mind functions. While it is impossible to stop this movement, through daily training we can slow down the film so we are seeing reality frame by frame and thus beginning to distinguish one moment, thought, or feeling from another. More important, we discover that just like a reel of film, with its tiny blank spaces between each image, a seamless and neutral continuity lies behind our chang-ing thoughts. Over time we can consciously shift our attention from the entertainment of passing images to the calm of the neutral back-ground.

Whether we're sitting in formal meditation, practicing a Yoga *asana*, or stuck in traffic, we can remind ourselves where and how we actually are. As we breathe in and out, we learn to attend to that which arises in one breath cycle and no more. Because the breath is one of the rare constants of life, we can use it as a metronome to delineate our experience. This is a very profound practice, and, while simple, it is not easy. The mind can drift with astonishing rapidity to past events, and before we know it we're thinking about what we should have said to so-and-so ten years ago (if only we'd had the presence of mind at the time) and what they would have said back and how we would have countered it. Before we know it, we've spent thirty minutes living out a full-scale soap opera in our heads with all the attendant feelings of rage and self-righteousness, not to mention the body tension that accompanies those feelings. Or we start fantasizing about the man sitting next to us at the meditation retreat, and by the end of the week we've gone through a courtship, romance, marriage, and divorce without even knowing his name. At times like this we can catch ourselves and say, "Well, the truth is, I'm just sitting here on this cushion breathing in and out." Or, "The truth is, I'm just in relaxation pose, breathing in and out." Or, "The truth is, I'm stuck in traffic, there's nothing I can do about it, and I'm breathing in and out." We can do this without beating ourselves up or being harsh critics. We can have a sense of humor about our phantasmagoric ramblings as we remind ourselves for the thousandth time that there's something more basic to attend to. Over time we catch ourselves sooner, we come back to the moment more easily, and we become less invested in entertaining ourselves with fantasy.

As we look deeper into this practice of dividing our experience into increments, we may discover the subtle ways in which we veer away from our immediate reality. While my students are holding a difficult Yoga posture, I often ask them what they are thinking. If we could script this inner monologue, it might sound something like this:

> I wonder when we're going to come out of this pose. I don't think I can hold my arms out to the side until the thirteenth breath. Everyone else seems to be doing better than me. I wish I

hadn't signed up for this class. I like the forward bends better. Boy, my arms are going to be sore tomorrow! I'll take a hot bath when I get home. I wonder if there's still any ice cream left in the freezer. If my roommate has eaten it all I'm going to . . .

Our experience becomes more and more difficult and increasingly dramatic as we try to steer around it. Meanwhile, if we could place ourselves more securely in the moment, we might find it quite pleasant and easily manageable. We might discover that while our arms feel tired, attention to our body might offer a better way to hold our arms up. When we learn to catch ourselves anticipating disasters that haven't yet happened or feeling righteous over past hurts, we can bring ourselves back to this moment and make our lives a whole lot simpler.

As we become more accustomed to this practice, we may start to notice that the breath is coming *from* somewhere. At the end of our exhalation there is a brief pause before the next breath arises. Curiously, this pause, of itself, is devoid of movement, thought, and sensation. The breath arises out of this pause and dissolves back into it. Gradually, as we train the mind to follow this progression, we develop a heightened appreciation for the value of this pause. It is the window into a field of silence that lies beneath the breath and is always present as a backdrop to the breath. Not only is this field of silence a backdrop to the breath, it is the backdrop to all our thoughts, feelings, and sensations. Through training our awareness to appreciate that there is something that does not move, we begin to practice the fifth limb of Ashtanga Yoga, *pratyahara*. Often translated as the withdrawal of the senses, in fact, *pratyahara* is more accurately translated as the movement of the mind toward silence rather than toward things. The practice of *pratyahara* prepares us to focus the mind on one thing at a time and, with training, to sustain this one-pointed focus under all conditions.

It should be said that there is nothing wrong with thinking, feeling, planning, or remembering. This is what the mind does. Thinking is not a problem. Many educated people who have spent their entire lives developing their minds balk at the idea of emptying the mind. If we imagine the mind as a neutral ground of awareness, it goes without saying that this ground of awareness will be richly embellished with all we've been taught, with our memories, and with our life experience. This too is not a problem. Some of those things may be very useful to us, like remembering our times tables, the meaning of words, or, more practically, our home address. The point of training the mind to return to this ground of awareness is to open to each moment from a fresh place. Then whatever we know from our experience that *is necessary to the moment* will percolate up from this neutral ground of awareness. This is how we can respond more creatively to life's challenges. If, however, we are always caught up in our fixed reference points and our contextual theories, we cannot respond from a fresh place. The breath is our most tangible way of gaining access to this effulgent resource. All we need do is follow one exhalation all the way down until the last whisper leaves the body, and there it is, that wonderful pause letting us know there is a neutral place from which to make a new beginning.

To the degree that the mind is preoccupied with memories of the past and fantasies of the future, that is the degree to which we cannot reside in the present moment. There is nothing intrinsically wrong with this stream-of-consciousness mind that bounces back and forth time traveling. However, in truth none of these past or future events exists. As long as our primary *participation* is with some other moment, our immediate experience will always be eclipsed. We go for a walk in the forest, and we're too busy thinking about our business problems to notice the freshness in the air and the smell of pine. We sit down to work at our desk, and we start to fantasize about that hike in the woods we have planned. When we're not busy being somewhere else, more often than not what we participate with is our past or future version of ourselves and our life. Instead of seeing how things actually are, we continue to see them as they once were or as we imagine they will be.

In questioning one of my students who comes to me with chronic back pain, I ask, "Are there any moments in the day when you do not feel this pain?"

"No, I feel this pain all the time."

Later as the class progresses, I ask, "How is your back feeling right now?"

"It feels good in this position."

"So there is a moment when you are not in pain."

"No, I have back pain all the time!"

Sometimes it can take many rounds of this kind of questioning for a person to realize how his experience has become fixed. As he begins to identify the moments when he is not in pain, he is then able to ask, "What am I doing right now that leads me to this pain-free experience? How exactly am I standing that gives me relief? At what point did I begin to feel ease?" And, "Can I enjoy this pain-free moment, however brief a respite?" As the mind becomes more aerated, it can begin to discern the details of an experience and to see that there is no experience that is permanent and intransigent.

And therein lies the key. For the moment we begin to participate fully with the present moment, we discover that with every breath we are changing. We start to notice that when we drink a cup of tea it is not the same at the beginning as at the end. The aroma is strongest when the tea is first poured. We can appreciate that moment. The first sip is the hottest. We appreciate that moment. As we get to the bottom of the cup, the tea is now cool. We appreciate that moment. Now we're left with the swirl of tea leaves in the bottom of the cup. We can take in that moment. Working with discrete increments of awareness gives us the ability to separate and define our day-to-day experience as multidimensional rather than the smear of consciousness that is the product of the untrained mind. Rather than all the colors running together in a blob, each and every color can stand out distinct and vivid. This lucid consciousness is characterized by a complete arousal of all the senses, which is at once blissful and satisfying. Often people turn to drugs or alcohol to notice the moment, recalling for years that wonderful LSD trip in which they reveled in the intricacies of a dandelion flower for hours on end. Yoga practice is a way to achieve lucidity in ways that are not destructive to ourselves or others.

The habitual untrained mind, however, rarely functions in this way. The untrained mind perceives things in a largely undifferentiated way, mashing together feelings, thoughts, and sensations into seemingly permanent forms and immutable conclusions. Past, present, and future fuse together in a drunken blur so that we cannot separate what was then and what is now. This ownership of a fixed identity prevents us from experiencing how we are changing. To discipline reality does not mean that we manipulate our perceptions to make them better or to control them. We discipline ourselves to notice that our reality *is* changing all the time, instead of forcing all our perceptions and experiences to conform to our fixed sense of things.

Our belief in ourselves as a fixed "I"-dentity can have devastating consequences. At the end of one intensive teacher training, the group gathered together to share their thoughts. One of the participants, Gloria, announced that she had decided to stop practicing Yoga and would definitely not be considering a future as a teacher because when she went inside she only experienced more intensely the grief of losing her son. This announcement was met with great shock by the other participants, who had observed that Gloria had a gift for teaching. In fact, Gloria seemed transformed when she was teaching and appeared to take great pleasure in instructing. She went on to tell us that she had been grieving deeply for many years, and she had come to accept that she would never, ever feel any different. Why do a practice that only reaffirmed this for her? Then one of her peers gently offered this question: "Were you happy before your son died?" Reluctantly, Gloria admitted she had been happy. "So, is this not proof that things can change?" Although we never knew the outcome for her, we all felt immensely saddened by her conclusions and how they might dictate her future.

When we bring ourselves back to the moment by steadying our breath, we ask the mind to sit up. If the mind were a dog, it should have its ears pricked. It doesn't matter what kind of practice we choose. We can use incremental awareness when we are making dinner, getting the kids ready for school, driving in hectic traffic, or holding a challenging Yoga posture.

What does this incremental awareness afford us? First of all, it allows us to reclaim our lives and the joy of everyday experiences. We become actualists instead of theorists or fantasists. We stop choosing for or against our experience on the assumption that it should somehow be different than it is. Once we drop these assumptions, we can start choosing to open ourselves to all of our experience, both pleasant and unpleasant. This choice allows us to become intimate with the breadth and depth of our humanity.

There is nothing heroic we need do in our Yoga practice to bring about this clear vision. Coming back to our breath increases our threshold for being with ourselves and the moment. Through this awareness we learn how to stay with ourselves and to stay with our practice. As we shall see in the chapter to come, this increased threshold for being with ourselves is the only way to gain access to our inner *atman*, our inner wisdom nature. Until we have developed this capacity we will be unable to establish our own personal Yoga practice. It is through such a practice that the design of our lives can reveal itself to us one breath at a time.

Chapter 10

The Inner Teacher

A certain day became a presence to me:
there it was, confronting me—a sky, air, light:
a being. And before it started to descend
from the height of noon, it leaned over
and struck my shoulder as if with
the flat of a sword, granting me
honor and a task. The day's blow
rang out, metallic—or it was I, a bell awakened,
and what I heard was my whole self
saying and singing what it knew: I can.

Denise Levertov,
"VARIATION ON A THEME BY RILKE"

Whether we are new to Yoga or have a long-established practice, the help and direction of a good teacher can accelerate our learning process and inspire our efforts. We may study with one teacher or many teachers, in one method or many methods. It's important, at least initially, not to dilute our studies by dabbling too widely, for it is usually only when the going gets rough that we start to penetrate to deeper levels of understanding. When we start to hit that wall or touch upon a core issue, staying with our teacher or a particular method of practice is vitally important lest we make a habit of always avoiding our sticking points. While having a teacher's guidance and outer direction is imperative at many stages of Yoga practice, we make a quantum leap when we begin to direct our own practice. That means practicing on our own.

What happens when we make that deep inner shift and arrive one morning on our mat or meditation cushion through our own volition?

At that moment we have begun to trust the inner guide that is leading us. We may not be able to see just yet where we are going, but we're willing to take a chance on ourselves. We might not lead ourselves through our practice with the same smooth assurance we experience when guided by a teacher, but through flexing our inner muscles we start to become more adept at doing so. We may not be certain that we're doing it right. We may not at first be as inspiring or as enthusiastic or as focused or as clear as our teacher, but increasingly we generate those same qualities. There is a measurable psychological and physiological shift when we self-suggest.[1] We become both the leader and the follower. At this point we have begun to join forces with our inner guide, our *antaryamin,* the manifestation of the Self within our own psyche. When we are in the process of internalizing the teacher and the teachings, we have begun to listen to what many of us intuitively know and refer to as our inner voice. Until we gain confidence in both listening to and following the promptings of this inner voice, we will always be looking for some outside authority to take care of us and tell us what to do.

Our inner guide can have many endearing qualities. He or she may be part parent, part cheerleader, part Mr. Tough Guy, part analyst, part wise sage, and part comedian. We may draw from our inner guide the qualities of a sister, an older brother, a father, a mother, a doting aunt, a wise grandparent, a transcendent deity, or a lover. As we get to know ourselves, we also get to know the qualities of our inner guide that we need to bring forth. If we are too lackadaisical, we may need to draw forth the stauncher, more directive guide, and if we are the sort of person who eats her banana with a knife and fork, we may need to find the guide in us that can help us to loosen up. Most important, our inner guide never gives up on us. No matter how bleak, hopeless, or pathetic our life appears to be, the inner guide still encourages us to stay with ourselves. This loyal and devoted allegiance is what we expect from our outer teachers but rarely offer ourselves.

I cannot emphasize enough the importance of making this shift toward self-practice for it is in this shift that things come together.

When we open ourselves to receive teachings, it is as if we have filled a huge pot with many nourishing ingredients. We fill it with raw onions and vegetables, lentils, ghee, and tasty spices. But none of these raw materials can be digested and assimilated until melded together by the heat of the fire and by slow cooking. When we start practicing on our own, it is as if we light a fire under ourselves. This fire brings the deep essence of the teachings to the surface. Just as a rich stew, once eaten and digested, becomes a part of our body, when we practice on our own the teachings become a part of us.

It can come as a surprise, then, to discover that only a tiny percentage of students who attend public Yoga classes and retreats practice on their own at home. The most frequently declared purpose for attending a retreat or workshop is to kick-start a flailing or nonexistent self-directed practice. So often we go to classes or retreats because we need the enthusiasm of the teacher to bolster us, and then we carry that enthusiasm home with us like a fragile parcel of gold dust. But our inability or unwillingness to exercise the potential power of our own inner teacher is like a hole in the matrix of our psyche, which, over the course of days and weeks, leaks that precious gold dust until our briefly bolstered enthusiasm has vanished. Now, of course, it's time to go to another class or retreat! But the one thing that is most likely to repair this gap in the psyche is practicing on our own. Through practicing on our own, we create a job for this inner guide: by sheer necessity some part of ourselves must step forward to fulfill the role we have created. As long as someone else is doing the job of directing, centering, disciplining, or encouraging, there will be no need for our inner guide to develop. Additionally, as we make the effort to practice on our own, we will inevitably come up against the cause of this psychic vacancy. We may discover that we have never felt worthy of our own attentions or that we make our own personal development a low priority. We may believe ourselves inept, incapable, and at worst, untrustworthy. It is rarely a case of simply needing more skills or technical knowledge to proceed. Rather, the job vacancy is there because we have not been willing or able to be an active participant in our spiritual practice. Certainly, teachers can help, and I am not suggesting that practicing on our own should replace ongoing instruction and mentoring. Everything we need from the teacher, however, is some part of ourselves that eventually we must draw forth from within ourselves. The fact that we recognize these qualities in the teacher can give us some clues as to the latent forces within us that need to be catalyzed.

One way we can begin this shift toward self-directed practice is to identify the qualities that we most admire and look for in our teachers. What has drawn us to them? When you have identified these qualities, look at the meaning these qualities hold for you and how you might embody these qualities yourself. In particular, look at some of the things you most take for granted. For instance, in all the time you have studied with your teacher, has she ever been late to class? Or ever judged or humiliated you? This quality of reliability and acceptance may give you a feeling of reassurance and steadiness. How might you offer yourself this same reliability and unconditional acceptance? Perhaps your teacher gives you his full attention and presence. You feel as if he is listening intently to your every word and question, responding to your every need. How could you offer yourself this same attentive awareness during your home practice and in so doing gain the courage to heed the promptings of your own inner guru?

In the best of all worlds a Yoga teacher models the behavior, attitude, and way of life that we would wish for ourselves. If the teacher embodies compassion and kindness in his or her being and communicates this awareness to us, the texture of our relationship to our self and to others will begin to mirror this loving quality of connectedness. But if our inner dialogue is unbalanced, we may seek out a teacher who will corroborate our own poor assessment of ourselves. Perhaps we are inwardly very judgmental or we have a tendency to be coercive or critical. Because these traits may be quite unconscious, we may unwittingly seek a teacher who exemplifies our inner judgment or forcefulness. A friend who had spent years trying to bolster her self-confidence went to see a teacher in India who upon seeing her declared, "You are *nothing!* You know *nothing!*" Her teacher proceeded over the course of three weeks to undermine any vestige of self-confidence she had acquired. After this bombardment of negativity, she came to realize she had found a teacher who merely amplified the violence she meted out to herself on a daily basis. Another student related how she was very impatient to progress and was drawn to work with a teacher who pushed his students hard. One day, seeing how restricted she was in her forward bends, he made a quick and forceful adjustment and tore her hamstring muscle. She realized then that she needed to find a more balanced approach to her practice. Her injury forced her to slow down and respect her limitations and to find a teacher who would respect them too.

If we can identify the tone, attitude, and content of our inner dialogue, we will be better equipped to find teachers who can help us find a kinder relationship with ourselves. For the greater part of my own early adulthood, I did not like my body, and much of my inner dialogue had to do with self-abhorrence. As a dancer I had great difficulty accepting my voluptuousness and longed to have the rail-thin, flat-chested bearing of my counterparts. To this end, I dieted and fasted obsessively. I can well remember the horror and shame of having a teacher stop a class and, pointing to my barely protruding abdomen, pronounce, "That is one of the most disgusting things I have ever seen!" This damaging comment, said only once, was not nearly as destructive as the silent barrage that took place for years afterward. As I began to recognize the inherent aggressiveness in this nonacceptance of my body, I also became drawn to study with a Yoga teacher who had a robust and curvaceous body. To be with someone who seemed to enjoy and completely embody her womanliness was a great eye-opener to me. Gradually I learned to accept my body as it was, and my inner dialogue about and toward my body became more celebratory.

When we find ourselves at a loss in guiding our own practice, we can begin to scrutinize the aspects of our inner guide that need development. We may find our practice frequently disrupted by the maelstrom of our emotions or the drama of our personal story. At times

like these it may be difficult to locate our inner guide, so caught up
are we in the particulars of our story. Further, we may mistake the
voice of our executive ego with that of our authentic inner guide so
that we become the blind leading the blind. If we are a ball of tension
or anger or sadness, we will be guided by an ego that is tense, angry,
or sad. Who is guiding whom?

The inner guide, however, always exists in the substratum of such
transitory phenomena, and when we need inner instruction we must
locate our minds here in order to receive information. One way of
distinguishing between the executive ego and the wisdom mind is that
information from the wisdom mind almost always presents the option we have least considered. It is usually a fresh and startling viewpoint, and because of this our insights can sometimes be a little scary.
Because we may not be skillful in locating this wisdom mind, especially if we are currently in the maelstrom of emotion, getting more
objective help from our teacher at such a time can be imperative. One
of my teachers, Ray Worring, had a remarkable ability to help me
shift my perception in order to see the bigger picture of a situation.
When I would call him in the throes of some emotional upset, enthralled by the importance of my drama, his friendly yet firm words
had a way of shifting my focus without putting me down while at the
same time opening a view to the light at the end of the tunnel. Since
his passing, I try to invoke that kind firmness in my own internal dialogue to help myself see past the immediate and fleeting feelings to a
broader perspective.

Another way we can work to internalize the teacher is to imagine
that we are the teacher "showing up" to teach the practicing student.
How might you feel if you knew others depended on you in this way
and you *had* to show up? Would you keep your appointment with
yourself to practice at a regular time and to bring your best focus to
your inner student?

For many years I actively imagined that each practice session was a
meeting with someone special. When we know we are meeting a loved
one, we take extra care dressing and grooming ourselves and we want

to bring the very best of ourselves forward. We make the room fresh and sparkling and take special care that it is beautiful and inspiring. Eventually that special someone we invite to our practice becomes us: we start to value ourselves so much that we want to treat ourselves in the best possible way. Albert Schweitzer, the great missionary, doctor, and musician, was often asked why he dressed in a formal suit to play the piano. Given his rough circumstances in the outer reaches of Africa, this behavior seemed at odds with common sense, not to mention the climate. He declared that when he played the piano he was meeting with God. How might each and every one of your home practice sessions be a meeting with a divine presence?

We can also learn a great deal about how to guide our own practice through becoming a better student. Many Yoga students expect a very high standard of behavior from their teachers but do not hold themselves to the same (or any) standard at all. Imagine if your teacher reclined back on his elbows as if watching a football game as he answered your questions. How would you feel if your teacher were caught up in her personal story or clearly bored or conducted the class while drinking her morning coffee and nibbling on a croissant? You would probably feel the teacher was not taking his or her role very seriously. But how often do we attend an intensive or retreat with no sense of what our role as a student is? When we begin to take a more active and conscious role as a student, we are moving in the direction of self-responsibility. When we make a special effort to bring our best energy, focus, and good cheer to our teacher (and more important, to our practice), we not only are expressing our appreciation for the teacher and the teachings, we are also beginning to show a deep respect toward ourselves. Taking a more conscious role as a student and examining one's behavior in this light can help us move from a passive dependence on the teacher to an active independence through the help of the teacher.

When I look back at the most important teachers in my life, I see that each offered me a significant contribution in my journey toward independence. While some offered a more intuitive approach to practicing, others taught me the value of discipline, routine, and persistence. Others taught me how to nut my way through a problem and creatively find my own solutions. My brief encounters with abusive teachers taught me as much as my long associations with good ones. I learned that I cannot learn in an atmosphere of fear and intimidation, nor do I respond to humiliation when it is used as a teaching tool. I learned how devastating it can be to have a teacher constantly criticize until one feels like nothing more than a temple of accumulated error. How disheartening it can be to struggle for the smallest improvement and not have one's teacher offer some praise. Through these less positive experiences, I learned how important it is to offer myself honest recognition when I have worked hard at something and to focus more on how far I have come rather than how much further I have to go. Through the many interactions with teachers, I have discovered what I respond to and what I do not respond to. This has been instrumental in discovering how to become my own best coach and how to structure my own practice.

However helpful any teacher has been, it is crucial that we not insert an outside authority within ourselves. When we do so, we tend to strive to have the experience we think we should have, and thus there is nothing we have discovered ourselves—nothing original or authentic. As Krishnamurti puts it, we become "secondhand people,"[2] having secondhand experiences. When we become the teacher's clone, we parrot information without the necessary inquiry and testing that will lead to healthy discernment. The most dangerous form of this replication process is when students give such unqualified allegiance to a teacher that they are led to rationalize and defend violent, abusive, or unwholesome behavior in the teacher. This is useful neither for the students nor for the teacher, who needs the students' doubts and challenges to continually assess the soundness of his or her understanding. To continually question and investigate a teacher or teaching is not a sign of disrespect but a sign that we are actively probing the soundness of information through the testing ground of our own experience and developing a healthy discriminative awareness. If an outside authority eclipses our own inner guide, we may lose this discriminative awareness and leave ourselves open to dire consequences.

Over the years I have counseled a number of students who were considering suicide rather than leave a teacher and method they knew to be harmful. In these extreme yet not uncommon student-teacher cult relationships, the teacher is internalized as a source of absolute certainty, and leaving the teacher or methodology means losing the security of this certainty. The teacher or outer authority has almost usurped the student's own inner guide. I say "almost" because inevitably the student experiences this takeover as a source of constant conflict. Even given this deep conflict, students caught in this trap may equate the alternative (leaving the teacher or organization) with being cast outside the village gates into outer darkness. The terror of facing the unknown is so great that many people will remain wedded to a teacher, method, or organization long after the marriage has proven itself barren. And because of this fear, the student may become the teacher's strongest defender, justifying and condoning unethical, egomaniacal, and even violent behavior, for if the teacher's authority is questioned, then, in essence, the student's own source of authority is on the line. When a student related to me that his teacher had kicked him in the head while he was in headstand, causing him to fall perilously, he defended his guru saying, "It was the best thing for me. I *needed* to be kicked in the head." Part of the reason people may remain for years in such a negative student-teacher relationship is that they feel they have no reliable inner guide with which to replace this outer authority. In many instances the teacher has actively and deliberately undermined the process of individuation by discouraging questioning of any kind, by negating or contradicting the student's perceptions, or by forbidding any creative deviation from a formal method. In such a student-teacher relationship there will never be a graduation ceremony. The student will remain forever infantilized in relation to the teacher. In such cases the person may require considerable support and counseling to begin the process of turning back toward and having renewed faith in his or her own inner wisdom.

At the other end of the spectrum, many Yoga practitioners have become self-proclaimed "workshop addicts," hopping from teacher to teacher gathering copious information that remains undigested and unintegrated. This is like repeatedly filling a glass with water without ever drinking from it. This dilettantism makes it almost impossible to internalize our own teacher, for we never allow ourselves to sustain any process long enough to do more than skim the surface. We don't learn how to dive deep with our teacher, and this makes it difficult to learn the skills to dive deep on our own. In this form of spiritual snorkeling, we limit ourselves to what can be seen from the surface. This is especially true if after many years of study we are still incapable of practicing on our own. At a recent teacher training conference, one of the students, Margot, was clearly making an important breakthrough. At the end of a very intense day of inquiry, I asked Margot's permission to give her my perception of her practice. I suggested to her that rather than increasing flexibility in her already hypermobile body, "containing her flow" would be a necessary skill not only in her physical practice but also in creating appropriate boundaries in her life. Margot related with some emotion that she had waited her entire life to have a teacher tell her this. It was clear from the emotional charge that accompanied this realization that Margot had touched on a core issue, important to every dimension of her life. So it came as some surprise when Margot approached me the next morning to tell me that she needed to switch to a different teacher. As I later discovered, she switched from teacher to teacher throughout the six-day conference, never letting any teacher get close enough to her to help her take the necessary next step.

If practicing without the help of a teacher feels like too big a leap, you might find a Yoga buddy or form a small group of fellow students and plan a regular time to practice together. Rather than having any one person lead the session, simply practice together, each doing his or her own practice with full concentration. Holding the intention of the practice helps others to hold their intention. Make an agreement that this is not to be a time for socializing. After your formal practice, make some time to discuss the issues or problems that arise in your individual practices and to share what you know with each other. If you are eager to catch up on each other's lives, plan to share a meal after practice. This will help you clearly delineate the formal practice from less formal social time.

If you are new to practice, give yourself realistic goals that you know you can achieve. Making a commitment to practice thirty minutes a day three days a week and keeping to it will be better than having grand plans to arise at 2 A.M. and practice for three hours each morning. If you set yourself unrealistic goals, you will inevitably abandon your personal practice and only reinforce the belief that you are incapable of such discipline. It takes time to build up a threshold for practicing on one's own, especially if you have not been accustomed to spending time by yourself. If you have great resistance to getting yourself on the mat, lure yourself by saying, "I'm just going to do three postures." After breaking the ice you will undoubtedly find you are eager to continue. Or if you are feeling really terrible, lure yourself by starting your practice with something particularly pleasant, such as a meditation you enjoy or a posture you find comforting. Consider handling yourself as you would a petulant child without getting into a battle of wills or being judgmental. When you start you may find yourself watching the clock. This is okay: as you become more immersed in your practice you will think less about how much more time you have to go and more about how little time you have to do your growing practice. Gradually you will look forward to your practice with real enthusiasm.

If you have an already well established practice, keep your practice fresh by incorporating new ideas. Use your time in class or at retreats to reinspire your efforts. Keep a notebook with you so that you can write down sequences that worked well for you, meditation practices you wish to try, and techniques that need further investigation. Take time to read books not only from the method you are studying but also from other Yoga traditions so that you can consider whether your own practice is balanced. You may have become too myopic in your approach or dismissive of other traditions. Or you may have developed one limb of practice while neglecting other limbs. As you become more refined in your personal practice, you may also need to seek a teacher who has greater depth or understanding. Most teachers realize when their students have outgrown them. Out of respect for the teacher who has helped you progress this far, take the time to thank your teacher for all she or he has done for you before moving on.

Whether you are a beginner or an advanced practitioner, when looking for a teacher, determine whether this teacher has his or her own strongly developed personal practice. Such a teacher will naturally stress the importance of self-practice. Teachers who believe that teaching class *is* their personal practice are likely using the students as their motivation for practice and have probably yet to develop a strong allegiance with their own inner *atman*. Their attention will at best be divided, and what they teach in class may be more determined by their own needs than by those of the students. Any teacher who claims that personal practice is no longer necessary has probably stopped learning and is ill prepared to foster an appetite for fresh inquiry in students. Most important, choose a teacher who clearly wishes to facilitate access to your own inner wisdom. Such a teacher will always find ways to throw you back on your own resources and challenge you to take command of your own life.

The kind of fruit we bear through practice, bitter or sweet, depends not only on what we do but also on how we do it. When you arrive on your mat and sit to begin your practice, you might pause for a moment and ask how you can cultivate a friendship with your self. How would your best friend speak to you at this moment? How might this person encourage you and bolster your confidence? How would she or he be honest with you in ways that did not leave you feeling diminished? If you are in pain, can you offer yourself the solace that a dear friend would generously give? If you are feeling joyful, can you be happy for yourself as a friend would be happy for you? The inner teacher has come to befriend you, and there is no part of you that is undeserving of this friendship. If our personal practice becomes a time of self-coercion and self-belittlement, each time we practice we leave a negative imprint and this makes it all the harder to come to the mat the next day. When we offer ourselves unqualified compassion, we start to make positive associations with our practice time. We become the kind of person we'd like to hang out with.

Finding a right relationship to oneself and to practice is the beginning of finding a right relationship to others and to the challenges of everyday life. We discover that this right relationship is a constant balancing act of effort and surrender, of concentrated focus and inclusive awareness, of firmness and gentleness. When we make a connection with our inner teacher, or *atman,* we are connecting with something larger than ourselves, and thus we begin to relinquish a sense of separateness. We discover that the world is inside us and we are inside the world. When we practice on our own, we create the conditions in which we are more likely to see that our happiness does not depend on something outside ourselves. An empty room, a mat, our body, and focused awareness—these are the simple means we use to open to the wholeness that waits within.

Chapter 11

Effort and Surrender

As much as you go out of all things that much, not more and not less,
God enters with all of his, insofar as you in all things completely give
up what is yours.

Meister Eckhart

When we begin our Yoga practice, or any significant endeavor for
that matter, it is unlikely we will get very far without making great effort. In these early stages of practice we need a little acceleration to
our efforts, like the running start we make on a bike before we go up
a steep hill. In the Yoga-Sutra Patanjali distinguishes between different kinds of effort. We are told that self-realization is imminent if
our actions are performed with ardor, enthusiasm, and sincerity and
that the more intense this passionate effort, the closer the goal
(I.2I–I.23). Yet immediately following this exposition on effort,
we're advised that effort and the spontaneous realization of oneness
are a contradiction in terms.[1] We can choose another option, and that
is to surrender to God. How do we reconcile these two seemingly
contradictory paths?

Anyone who has tried to think their way out of a difficult problem
realizes at some point that the mind can take us only so far. This is
true also of effort and the use of will. When we begin, there is a
short-term, ebullient kind of effort that is absolutely required. The
first push down on the bike pedal is always the hardest because we
have not yet built up acceleration. When we learn anything—playing
an instrument or speaking a new language—there is always an initial
period in which we must break through our ineptness. No matter

how clever we are, we cannot leapfrog over this initial period in which we may be all fingers and toes. In the long-term view of a life practice we must still use effort, but our effort will be of a different kind. Since we have established our capacity for volition, our effort may now be in relinquishing that part of the effort that is not possible for us to do. When we refuse to surrender up that part of the work that cannot be traversed through will, it is like continuing to pedal our bike even though we're now headed downhill. In the beginning of our spiritual quest we can accomplish nothing without effort. But at a certain point in our journey we can accomplish nothing more through effort. Through effort we come to step into a stream that can carry us. When we begin to let this current carry us, gradually the person who is making the effort needs to take a backseat. At this juncture we spontaneously shift from an "effort to be" to effortless being.

Ramana Maharshi, the great jnana[2] Yoga adept, was said to have reached his own self-realization not through effort but by spontaneous awakening. Born in India, Maharshi led a rather uneventful life until his teens. Then one day he "suddenly experienced an intense fear of death, which prompted him to picture his own cremation and dissolution. This imaginative exercise led to his discovery of the Self beyond the physical body. In this way he became Self-realized at the age of sixteen."[3] Maharshi described the mind as like a stick used to stir a funeral pyre: eventually the stick itself is subsumed by the fire. Yet being subsumed does not imply being passive or complacent, nor does it exonerate us from making an effort. His recorded dialogues with students in the years that followed his spontaneous enlightenment centered on the truth of oneness and, as it appeared to him, the irrefutable logic of indivisibility. But in reading the questions and responses of his disciples, one senses an enormous chasm between what is ironically self-evident to Maharshi through his direct experience and what cannot be grasped by the student's mind without this prior experience.[4] It is like the catch-22 of trying to establish credit for the first time. You can't get credit without credit. One cannot realize oneness without first experiencing oneness. Or, as the Yoga-Sutra commentator Vyasa states, "Yoga can only be known by Yoga. Yoga manifests through Yoga." It is a conundrum with seemingly no answer.

Maharshi recommended two basic approaches to self-realization: either completely surrender to a higher power (whatever form that higher power takes), or through your own effort investigate the cause of suffering and ponder the question: "Who am I?" Like a dog following the scent of his master through thicket and field, following this question by using thorough investigation and contemplation was guaranteed to gradually penetrate the layers of false identities and bring one home to the Self. By eliminating illusory identities, we gradually discover who we are not and thus come closer to knowing who we are. These supposedly alternate paths contain and lead inexorably to each other. Like a river that forks and branches, creating two separate channels, both inquiry and surrender arise from the same source and are compelled by the same passionate question.

How we find a balance between self-volition and this place of surrender is unique to each individual and certainly influenced by our particular predilections, constitution, family upbringing, education, cultural conditioning, and if you believe in such things, past lives. For the most part, the mind, convinced of its own preeminence, must now be thoroughly convinced of its limitations. *The mind has to wear its "self" out.*

Many of us come to this place of surrender after exerting every possible effort to achieve something and still finding ourselves well short of our goal. When we come to this place the only thing left to do is to surrender to the mystery of our own destiny and to trust in something we cannot yet fathom from the limited perspective of the little self. We might be battling with some ethical dilemma, and we've made lists of pros and cons, but nothing brings us closer to knowing which way to go. Then we head out for a walk, and our mind goes blank, and after a few hours the solution appears.

Early in my teaching career I had an experience that profoundly shaped my relationship to the practice of surrender. In the late eighties the small classes conducted in my Victorian house in San Francisco began to draw the attention of the landlord, who regretfully notified me that for legal reasons the classes must cease. For months I searched for a new place in which to teach, calling every church, school, and meeting place that might be suitable. Finally, having no luck, I resorted to walking streets and lanes and saw For Rent signs, but to no avail. I came home one evening particularly disheartened and had a frank discussion with God. Clearly he (or she) did not want me to continue to teach. Clearly this was a sign that I should move on to something else. In complete resignation, I decided that I would give up all attempts to find a studio, and if the powers that be wanted me to teach, well, they could find me a place in which to do it. The next morning the phone rang: "I hear you are looking for a place to teach." This experience did not diminish my sense that all my efforts had in fact been necessary. Just because someone like Einstein happens upon his greatest insights while riding a bike doesn't mean the years of study, thought, and analysis that preceded those insights were worth nothing. The two practices go together.

One can see the relationship between effort and surrender even in the simplest practice such as *Savasana*, or Corpse Pose. So, for the sake of anchoring our discussion in practice, imagine for a moment that you have just entered the pose of complete relaxation. You lie on your back like a corpse, as you will at the end of your life. This is a dress rehearsal for the ultimate relinquishing of the body, with the good news that it is only a temporary exercise. When you begin *Savasana* it is necessary to guide yourself mindfully into relaxation. If the mind is not taking part in this active guiding process, you are likely to drift off into an endless stream of internal chitchat. At this point in the practice the mind sets limits, and we agree not to move about, not to participate in thoughts, feelings, and sensations, and to progressively relax each and every part of the body. At a certain stage of relaxation, the mind becomes still and the experience of quiet consciousness dominants. When we become adept at this process, we relax our grip so completely that we enter a suspended state that is without normal discursive thought. Within this potent stillness there is wealth of information that we cannot access through the normal channels of the habitual mind. The mind has thus served its purpose. It is like a ticket that has gotten us onto the train: we don't need to keep holding the ticket for the rest of the journey.

Now look back at the times when your practice of *Savasana* was deep and refreshing. If you have ever carefully made note of this, you may have seen a connection to the effort during the practice that preceded *Savasana*. If you spent the practice flouncing around, eyeing the dust balls under the sofa or picking your toenails, it's likely you had great difficulty entering *Savasana*. The mind unexercised remains full of piss and vinegar. So when we come to *Savasana* we circle our toes, readjust our blankets, and cycle through some of our old internal tapes just for good measure. Like a person who has never lived, when we come to our death we are filled with regrets and now cannot die well either. If the mind has been exercised through one-pointed concentration throughout the practice, the mind then readily welcomes the opportunity to take a backseat, as if to say, "Whew! I've done my job, now you take over." And this "you" that takes over is the consciousness of the Self. Here we can see that effort and surrender are mutually dependent states.

Whether we are able to relinquish struggle in our lives has a great deal to do with our relationship to both effort and surrender. We can have many responses to these two forces. The first, but not necessarily the most common, response, is the neurotic one. A person with a neurotic relationship to these forces has chosen neither effort nor surrender. She cannot make an effort to change her situation, and she cannot surrender to it. Most tellingly, she cannot relinquish attachment to even the most miserable of states. Caught in a litany of complaint and blame (usually about other people, and conditions supposedly out of her control), the neurotic neglects to step up to the plate even when she is the only member on the team left to play. This person fails to understand that some things *are* under her control and that blind surrendering up of self-responsibility does not lead to happiness. We have all been this person at one time or another. Perhaps the most common way this condition plays itself out is in our intimate relationships. We may see our unhappiness as contingent on someone else changing while never being willing or able to see our own responsibility in making choices. We are unhappy because we live with someone who is abusive, but we do not see our unhappiness as a result of our failure to choose an alternative. Or we might complain about a health condition when we've been unwilling to actively do our share in improving our health. However this neurotic ruse manifests, it is based on an inability to be honest with ourselves. Whether we're dealing with ourselves or another, withdrawing self-pity, sympathy, or support for this dishonesty is one step toward extricating ourselves from our own complicity in creating our own unhappiness.

Many of us start our Yoga practice as neurotics. When Emily came to a screening interview for a special-needs class for people with back problems, she brought with her a long list of therapies and therapists that, as she put it, "had failed her." Her referring physical therapist related that Emily's unwillingness to do any home exercises or to address her weight issue made improvement unlikely. It was clear that Emily had played the same game with all her doctors. I tried a different tactic.

"So when does the first class start?" she asked, absentmindedly looking out the window.

"I'm afraid I don't think you'll be suitable for our program."

"What do you mean!" she said, jumping to attention.

"Well, I could not in all honesty guarantee that you would see any improvement unless you were willing to do thirty minutes of practice each day in between the scheduled classes."

"Oh," she said with a conspiratorial glint in her eye, "I'm not likely to do any exercises at home."

"Well, I'm very sorry, but I wouldn't want to waste your time or mine. Perhaps you should think about whether you are serious about improving your back condition and call me in a week."

Given these new conditions, Emily did eventually decide to attend the class, and for the first time she noticed an appreciable reduction in pain. We insisted that she chart her daily progress so she could see the clear relationship between the days she practiced and her reduced pain levels. Unfortunately, there are many people like Emily who never extricate themselves from their own self-induced misery. And unfortunately, there is often little that others can do to help. With a neurotic response, we often have an extremely low tolerance for any process that does not come easily. Because of this low tolerance for difficulty, it is best to break down a task into manageable increments and in the process gradually build up a threshold for the challenge of learning.

Then there is halfhearted effort. If we've made a halfhearted effort, some residue will be left from our action. When we know in our heart that we haven't put our best foot forward, the residual trace of this incomplete action niggles at us. It lingers within us, becoming self-judgment, disappointment, or regret. The accumulation of these residues can make it difficult to relax because some part of us compulsively revisits the past to do it over again. This doing it over again can take many forms, from obsessing to rehashing to an ongoing sense of urgency caused by the weight of things undone. When such reluctance is present, it usually means that a part of us is ambivalent, and this part of us, however small, can act like a thousand-pound weight that we drag behind us. As anyone who has ever vigorously cleaned their house will know, whole-hearted effort takes half the time and is twice the fun. For the halfhearted, discovering the exhilaration and benefits of full-fledged commitment can be a strong remedy for rallying energy and directing it toward a purpose. Spending time around others who are fully engaged and focused can be one way to learn the necessary attitudes and ethics required for whole-hearted living.

For some, however, the relationship between effort and surrender is more onerous. If you are a perfectionist for whom surrender is always contingent on things completely outside your control, you may never allow yourself to enjoy the ride. For such a "conditional perfectionist," happiness rests on certain conditions being met. Even when the mind has given itself completely to the task, when all that can be done has been done, there is such an attachment to an ideal outcome that it becomes impossible to let go. For such a person, the surrender may be in letting go of the attachment to what is perceived as the correct and just outcome. For instance, I have spent many of my twenty-eight years of Yoga practice dealing with various forms of back pain. This often comes as a great surprise to others, who perceive me as the epitome of physical agility, but genetics and old injuries combined with the rigors of computer work and heavy lifting make it necessary for me to give enormous care to my spine. In my early years of practice, a good day, a day worthy of happiness, was a day without back pain. Regardless of how many hours I had spent on the mat, I could define myself and my success only in terms of lack of physical pain. The trouble was, the pain rarely left. Greater effort in practice didn't always correlate to less pain. It took many frustrating years of practice to realize that this was the case not only with physical pain but with *everything!* No amount of practice in the morning would guarantee that life would be a bowl of cherries that day. Even though you have dotted your *i*'s and crossed your *t*'s, the battery might still be stolen from the car, the kitchen drain might clog before a big dinner party, and the clearest communication might lead to a horrible standoff with your spouse.

If you are a person with conditional perfectionist tendencies, it will be important to make agreements with yourself. For instance, I might agree that five days a week I will do the postures that strengthen my back, even if these are not my favorite ones. But it will be just as important for me to have an agreement that if my strategy fails that I surrender to rather than struggle with the outcome. If I can honestly say I have done what I can, then I can relinquish the struggle and attempt to find an accepting relationship with pain. In the same way, you might be in the process of psychotherapy or counseling, trying to resolve some deep conflict that has plagued you. While it will be important to give yourself to this inner work, it's equally important to be at peace about the outcome on a moment-to-moment, day-to-day basis. "I have done what I can do, and if I am still sad or angry or jealous, then so be it." Can I develop an accepting relationship to a less-than-ideal outcome? This unconditional acceptance is an important part of any spiritual education, or we will continue to struggle when struggle is futile.

Beyond the conditional perfectionist is the "impossible perfectionist," for whom no outcome or accomplishment, however ideal, is satisfying. He has attained the thirty-minute headstand and is now aiming to do it with no hands. Such a person is always moving the finish line. Can you imagine how a child would respond to such a learning strategy? And what happens when we offer ourselves no reward or acknowledgment for even our finest efforts? Effort in this case is being used to eclipse fear. The fear of relinquishing control may be so ingrained that just at the moment when we could be relaxing, we are setting up a fire hoop with bigger and hotter flames to jump through. Fortunately, like the consumer who has amassed a lifetime of toys only to discover he is still not having fun, the impossible perfectionist's effort will eventually lead to a conclusion. After attaining the thirty-minute headstand without hands and practicing this austerity diligently for years, he is likely to conclude, "Is this all there is?" By eliminating what cannot be achieved through effort, it is possible to get closer to the mystery of what can be realized only through surrender. The path of the impossible perfectionist is, however, a harsh one.

Judith Lasater, Yoga teacher and author of *Living Your Yoga,* has a wonderful phrase for those of us who never let up. She suggests saying silently or out loud, "I am attempting something difficult, and I appreciate myself for trying." Or, "I have just done something difficult, and I appreciate myself for trying."[5] Now watch the dialogue that follows. When you succeed, when you falter, or when you fail, what is the tone of this dialogue? Is it harsh and dismissive, or is it gentle and encouraging? Listening to this inner dialogue can be enormously useful in assessing our relationship to our self and how this inner relationship may color our interactions with others.

Another way of practicing this acceptance and relinquishing is to say silently or out loud, "This is as good as it gets." We can look at the telltale oil leak on the garage floor and give up fighting. Even when we think we are experiencing the worst possible outcome, we can try on this "good as it gets" philosophy. And even if this feels like a big leap, it's worth faking it to see what happens. If nothing else, it will develop your sense of humor, which in itself is a sign of spiritual progress. I will never forget the astonishment on a friend's face when after he had related the tragic deaths of two of his family that day, his spiritual teacher replied with gentle yet sincere enthusiasm, "This is a wonderful opportunity for you!" This extraordinary statement simply shattered my friend's concept of how he could respond to such a loss. When we can say this is as good as it gets and mean it, we are saying that nothing in our experience needs to be excluded and nothing in our experience is unworthy of our acceptance. We stop judging our experience, saying, "I'll take this one but not that one." We stop wrestling with our experience based on what should or should not have happened.

Coming to this encompassing acceptance is one of the most blessed gifts of Yoga practice. When we cease to identify ourselves with things outside our control and when we cease to wrongly attribute our success or failure to these things, we are well on the way to finding a place of inner ease that *no one* and *no thing* can take away from us. Interesting things happen when we give up struggling with a situation or problem outside of our control. When we stop trying to fix something that will not and cannot be fixed and we accept it just as it is, we liberate our energy. All the energy that we have poorly invested in struggle is now freed for other purposes.

One of the people who has greatly inspired my understanding of surrender is an extraordinary woman, Kathy Appel, who hosts me in her home during my teaching visits to Kelowna, Canada. Now in her forties, she became blind due to diabetes in her twenties soon after the birth of her first child. It is hard to fathom how overwhelmingly frightening this experience must have been. But what I find most amazing about Kathy is her genuine cheerfulness and the obvious pleasure she takes in the simplest things. Her condition has not stopped her from traveling regularly around the world, such is her joy in exploring new places. One day, while out on a walk with her and her equally impressive guide dog, Shade, I asked how she had come to this inner happiness. Given her condition, didn't she find navigating her way through strange streets on her foreign ventures just a little scary? "Well, you see," she smiled, "the worst has already happened! What is left to fear?" Accepting her blindness as a given was obviously a crucial step in coming to this courageous state of being. We might say that she didn't have any other choice. Her blindness is irreversible. But, in truth, most of what happens to us moment to moment is also irreversible. If we could imagine our present condition were as irreversible as my friend's blindness, what would our relationship be to our difficulties?

Where is this surrender leading us? Why is it important? As we've already seen, the mind that creates a problem is not the same mind that can solve the problem. The mind that sees itself as a separate "I" cannot at the same time relinquish this "I." Everything and everyone will be processed through the lens of this "I" and conceptualized in relation to it. It's like having fingers covered in ink. You get dressed in the morning, and your clothes get covered in inky fingerprints. You shake hands with a new friend, and you've left your inky mark. By the time the day is over, you just can't figure out where all those black marks came from and why everything you own and everyone you know looks inky. Then you look down at your hands and realize you're the culprit!

We may temporarily need this "I" that desires and longs for happiness to propel our very efforts. But at a certain point in the journey we can't go any further until we drop our "I"-dentity. The mind that is defined by "I" is also limited by "I." It cannot by definition perceive and experience what is limitless. So like a physicist struggling to crack the code of the universe, at a certain point we have to "relax our conventional conceptual constraints."[6] This relaxing into consciousness makes available to us a new and altogether different view of reality. The energy that we have been using to maintain the boundaries of the mind and use the mind as a guiding force is now liberated to serve the unbinding of consciousness. When the walls of the mind begin to crumble in this way, a whole new world opens to us. The stick has begun to be subsumed by the fire.

Many of us experience glimpses of this unboundedness. This can happen spontaneously, but more frequently it happens when we've been worn down to such a degree that we haven't the energy to keep defending the fortress. Once, after being very ill for nine months and at the end of my tether, I lay down for a brief nap only to discover myself sitting bolt upright a few moments later. An intense, indescribable rush of energy accompanied by a thunderous sound moving through my spine and out the top of my head had awakened me. When I related this to my spiritual mentor, he noted with dry disinterest, "Oh, yes, that sounds like an experience of kundalini." "But why in a dream!" I countered, exasperated. "Well, if you'd been awake you would have stopped yourself!" When we relax into consciousness, we avail ourselves of new information that the little me could not have imagined—or allowed. Yoga is a technology for making this random, tenuous connection with the Self an everyday experience.

How do we loosen the straitjacket of the mind and open to this realization of indivisibility? There is a certain point in the spiritual quest where the mind lies down and the heart takes over. Some people call this new locus their instinct, core awareness, or simply *knowing*. In yogic understanding, the heart *is* the Self. There is a sensate quality to this shift from the mind as locus to the heart as the instrument of inquiry. This shift is felt rather than understood and has the sensate quality of falling back, as one would fall back into the warm arms of a loved one. Our sense of self dilates like the pupil of the eye and begins to encompass everything. The gaze begins to soften, and we start to see from an internal vision. We may continue our spiritual search, but we have now narrowed the search to something within ourselves.

This shift is exemplified in the poem of the fifteenth-century Indian poet and mystic Kabir:

> The small ruby everyone wants
> has fallen out on the road.
> Some think that it is east of us,
> other west of us.
> Some say, "among primitive rocks,"
> others, "in the deep waters."
> Kabir's instinct told him it was inside,
> and what it was worth.
> And he wrapped it up carefully
> *in his heart cloth.*[7]

This shift of locus does not mean we no longer encounter difficulty or struggle. Everything does not automatically go swimmingly just because we're going about it in the right way. I am always amused when I tell people I am a Yoga teacher and they inevitably say, "Oh, that must be so relaxing for you!" In truth, life has never rendered up so many challenges. Gradually, though, as one lives more and more from the core of one's being, there is no one left to struggle. Struggle happens, but there is no one claiming ownership of the experience. We become transparent to experience, in the same way that wind moves through the branches of a tree. It is not that we no longer feel pain, it is that we no longer cling to it in such a way that our pain becomes suffering. And most important, our experience serves to soften the heart so that we are able to embrace even the most difficult experience.

David Godman, editor of *Be as You Are: The Teachings of Sri Ramana Maharshi*, describes what happens when we relinquish this ownership of experience: "When self-inquire reaches this level there is an effortless awareness of being in which individual effort is no longer possible since the 'I' who makes the effort has temporarily ceased to exist."[8]

As the sense of "I-ness" diminishes, we gradually develop a knack for welcoming experience with impartiality. One witnesses all experience as if it is happening to someone else. When I began working with the practice of impartiality, I imagined that it would cause a kind of coldness or remoteness from life's experience, which seemed an undesirable goal. One day, after wheeling my supermarket cart into the parking lot and looking unsuccessfully for a few minutes for my car, I heard myself say, "Oh, *her* car has been stolen!" Standing in the parking lot, I observed this impartial witness considering, in a very good-humored way, what to do with all her groceries. Looking down at the melting ice cream, a quiet openness bordering on wonderment filled me. I understood at that moment that impartiality is central to finding ease in life and that impartiality leads not to a deadening of spirit but to an enlivening that occurs when we are open to outcome. When we come to this place of relinquishing struggle, the heart, now centered within itself, can offer us an immense compassion and acceptance that the mind cannot know.

Chapter 12

Trusting the Mystery

Your task is to love what you don't understand.
Rainer Maria Rilke

When we're not sure, when we're filled with doubts or in the throes of despair, when we've tried as hard as we can, or when we're clinging to a bad situation because we're too afraid to let go, Patanjali gives us one simple solution. As often as is necessary, bring the mind back to a single focus (Yoga-Sutra 1.32). And what is this single focus? Focus, he tells us, on the absolute certainty of your connection with life no matter how unfathomable this life may be. This is not a hard thing to do, of course, when everything is going our way and the mystery is filled with positively good news and good fortune. It doesn't occur to us to wrestle with the whys and wherefores of this present happiness. Yet when things don't go our way, and there's seemingly no explanation for our current run of bad luck, our first tendency may be to contract or, alternately, to run toward anything that might offer us a sense of safety. Patanjali tells us that we don't really have freedom until we have a third choice: something between the obvious polarities of attraction and aversion, holding on to or pushing away. Turning our attention back to our center is a way of standing in between these two polarities and opening ourselves to a third option. This third option opens us to creative solutions, to possibilities our little self isn't able to generate, and puts us squarely where we might see how best to navigate out of a sticky situation.

When we focus the mind and bring it back to center, we find a place of spaciousness. It is here we have enough room to let the mystery we call life live itself through us. By bringing our attention back to the transparent nature of consciousness, we can experience bad things without feeling so much need to contract, to hold on, or to run away. Turning toward this mystery, however, can feel like jumping from the frying pan into the fire. The very largeness of life can overwhelm us. For this reason, when we hit a roadblock in the path, Patanjali advises us to stay with one method, one practice, and one focus because this one-pointedness will lead us inexorably to our center and the spaciousness of this mystery. It is through trusting the ineffable nature of our center that we can find the deepest possible security.

Theory and practice, unfortunately, are two very different things. When our retirement funds have just disappeared with a crashing stock market or our partner is diagnosed with cancer, theory doesn't give us much of a cushion. This is why we practice. We practice finding our center and staying in our center in the hothouse conditions of practice so that when push comes to shove, we will know where to turn.

Driving in the car late one night, I switched on the radio to stay awake. The only station on the dial featured one of those charismatic preachers ranting and raving about faith. In spite of my cynicism, I decided to listen for a while. Overwrought delivery aside, this preacher had a very good point to make. He told his audience, "If you spend five minutes in prayer every day and five hours in front of the TV, which do you think you'll turn to in times of trouble?" He said that having faith in the mystery of God and of life was like always having a fatherly or motherly presence with us. "When you have that presence with you, like a little child walking with his parents, you won't be scared by even the biggest and nastiest dog."

Sitting in meditation a few days later, I found myself distracted and worried by, among other things, two seriously ill parents, a recent announcement of bankruptcy by someone who owed me a large sum of money, and impending construction of a new home. After a few minutes of stream-of-consciousness worrying, I heard a small voice suggesting, "Let go." "Let go of what?" "Everything." "Everything?" "No—every thing." Opening my eyes, I looked out at the panoramic view of ocean and sky that can be seen from my small hillside cottage in New Zealand. Birds diving in the breeze, the branches of trees moving, the sun glistening on the surface of the water. Let go, this voice seemed to be saying, of every thing that is not the mystery itself.

It's easy to trust in the mystery when everything is going our way. This is why it's prudent to use these happy times to practice bringing the mind back to center. Practicing in good times lays a strong ballast in our boat so that when the going gets rough we can skillfully keep ourselves upright. This is exactly why Patanjali tells us, when you're in the middle of a storm, stay with one method. This is not the time to be wishing you were somewhere else or thinking about trying out some new sailing techniques you've only just read about. Why does Patanjali give us this advice? Because it is exactly at these moments that we are excruciatingly close to discovering the truth of how reliable and tangible and *real* this mysterious center is.

If we haven't formed the habit of staying in our center, when things get rough we will run in ever-widening circles away from or around our center. We may be more comfortable with our histrionics and with the drama born of such neurosis than we are with the simple practice of staying centered. When we're pacing the periphery looking for something to cling to, the mind hardens and the heart begins to clench in fear. In such a state of contraction, it is just as impossible to let go as it is to open up to the potential freshness of the next moment. As the saying goes: If you are very, very careful, nothing bad or good will ever happen to you. While pain is inevitable, suffering is not. By clinging to our existentialist viewpoint, we take a bad situation and make it worse by trying to wrestle it to the ground, like a person desperately trying to stop the incoming tide. Unconsciously, we may believe that this clinging and holding on for dear life is our only choice. Patanjali gives us another choice and declares: Let go.

There may be other causes for our tendency to live always on the periphery of our center, always distrusting the mystery that is implicit in life. *We may have a paralyzing fear of our own insight.* When we touch base with our center and get quiet, we begin to sense what we need to do, and maybe this is not the comfortable life we've carefully mapped out for ourselves. We may be working as a retail clerk, but our mystery beckons us to return to art school. We may hope for a life of luxury, but our mystery tells us to travel to West Africa and work in the Peace Corps. We may find these insights a damned nuisance because they seem so *inconvenient.* And these insights, offering new and spacious possibilities, seem so scary relative to the known, even if the known is a life of discontent.

When Helena, a strikingly attractive young woman, came to her first women's Yoga retreat, she seemed the picture of happy youthfulness. As the retreat wore on, she began to share her reservations about her current relationship with a man twice her age. He had already indicated no desire to have children (an option she wished to keep open), and his all-consuming career made her a marginal priority, scheduled into the remaining slots of his work calendar. He had already stated that although he thoroughly enjoyed her company, "she could leave at any time," reinforcing her feelings of superfluousness. Helena began to relate how many of her relationships bore this pattern of her being an ornament for her partner. Late one evening while making finishing touches to her mask (a telling blank white face with a sparse sprinkling of sequins), Helena confided, "I knew after a day, perhaps the first night. Something in me said, Get up and get out. I just knew it wasn't going to work. But almost immediately another voice took over and I stayed." Through the mentoring of older women retreatants who, through their own spiritual practice, had gained the courage to stand on their own, Helena began to see that she had many options. As days of meditation, *asana* practice, and quiet self-reflection continued, Helena showed a growing confidence about stepping out of this unsatisfactory situation and stepping back into her own center of gravity. Months later she sent me a change-of-address notice, saying she had returned to school to pursue the studies she had spoken about so passionately.

Some of us come to this central inner reference out of a gradual process of inner tempering. Through practice we become strong enough to know what we know and to bear the paradoxical consequence of freedom. Most of us, however, come to this place when we reach a point of inner desperation and, like Helena, have come to see that all our old tricks and self-deceptions haven't worked. Others of us simply become so tuckered out pacing the periphery of our center that we finally arrive at the center out of sheer resignation. Still others are brought kicking and screaming by life circumstances. How we come back to center doesn't really matter, but it matters terribly that we do.

What do we find when in the center? When we move our awareness beneath the transitory parade of likes and dislikes, thoughts and fears, we return to the original stillness of the mind. This central hub is referred to variously as the essence, pure consciousness, primordial mind, original mind, wisdom mind, or simply our natural mind. Most important, within this natural mind lies a domain of information we cannot find through the normal channels of our habitual, rational mind.[1] Tuning in to this natural mind is rather like tuning in to a radio frequency where the broadcast is completely silent and the transmission is felt by the heart rather than heard by the ear. We can realize this naturally calm mind in many ways—through meditation, through ethical living, through service, through being in nature, or through association with peaceful people. The natural mind is characterized by an all-pervading peacefulness and an unbounded spaciousness. It is not that this quiet stillness and spaciousness is somewhere else and we need to leave our experience to find it. Rather, our thoughts, feelings, and sensations are permeated by this spaciousness. Everything we experience arises out of this spaciousness and dissolves back into it.

This natural mind is the feeling we have when we're walking in the woods and the mind suddenly ceases its normal chatter. At such moments all the senses become present to the basic process of living. The mind becomes large, the world becomes large, and we become large. We take in the scent of pine, the crack of the branch underfoot, the subtle hue of moss, and the dampness in the air, and we feel a deep sense of belonging to every thing that is living itself through us. We see the infinite reach of the sky and the unimaginable depth of the ground we're standing on and realize we *are* that. When the normal discursive mind moves into the background, the natural mind takes a foreground position, and it is from this mind that some of our most lucid insights arise. We may spontaneously see the solution to the problem we've been wrestling with. Or our heart becomes serene in the face of no solution. When we are tuned in to the natural mind, we find we have access to a source of information that brings us closer to the mystery of life. We get a sense that this Christmas we should visit our parents, and sure enough by the new year one of our parents has passed away. We sense, without having to understand our senses, that someone is worthy or unworthy of our trust. When we get better at this, we start being able to follow our insights and intuitions without having money-back guarantees up front.

Coming back to center and relaxing into the mystery is the beginning of relinquishing our last stronghold: our belief that we are small and separate. When a student I'll call Robert began taking Yoga classes, he appeared very guarded but nonetheless was seeking some respite from the stress of his corporate career. Like many people, he found the relaxation at the end of class, called *Savasana*, or Corpse Pose, the most enjoyable part of practice. At first Robert would lie in *Savasana* with his eyes open, darting from place to place, as if his mind were hovering a few feet above his body. After many months Robert began to let his hair down, revealing a person of genuine warmth and humor. One day, following a long guided meditation on Corpse Pose, I noticed that Robert had entered a profoundly deep state of relaxation. Just at the moment when the room became absolutely still, he suddenly sat bolt upright, something he later described as "a movement beyond my conscious awareness." He stared wide-eyed around the room as if he had seen a ghost. "I really thought," he explained later, "I thought I was losing it. I thought I was going to die."

The Yoga-Sutra tells us that the fear of death is instinctual and inborn no matter how learned we may be (2.9). This unconscious and perfectly normal fear is the fear of relinquishing what we mistakenly take to be our *only* self and relaxing into the consciousness of this larger Self. Relaxing into this larger experience of ourselves *as* consciousness can be perceived as a death of an old way of life. We may know that there is some larger life to which we wish to belong, but it is an unknown quantity relative to the familiarity of our smaller life. What we fail to see is that this separate identity is actually a very lonely and shut-off place. It is like living in a house with all the curtains drawn and all the windows shut. Opening ourselves to be this larger Self doesn't mean we have to burn down our house. It just means we need to open the doors and windows and let in some light and air.

If we perceive ourselves as small and limited, we will perceive this vastness as a threat to our security. Even as we are dismantling one form of our identity, we may be in the process of erecting a new inner scaffolding upon which our new sense of self can rely. And this identity-making, security-seeking process will always fail if what we identify with is outside our center. For instance, we may have relied on our identity as a successful businessman or businesswoman, and without this we feel insecure. Perhaps we grow to question this identity, but even as we are loosening our grip of reliance on this identity, we may be forming another. Now we are an adept hatha yogi or yogini, able to do extraordinary postures. We may become just as bound up in our identity as a spiritual Yoga person as we were with our corporate persona. We once again become bounded by this new persona. The executive ego is always invested in perpetuating its own supremacy and not orchestrating its own demise. The life of the Self, on the other hand, is characterized by awe, mystery, and open-endedness. And while we might find living in awe, mystery, and open-endedness rather nice for an evening at the theater, living our whole life this way may feel like a tall order.

In Yoga practice, we consciously increase our threshold for living at this level of intensity without fracturing. This is one reason it is so important to stay continually with the practice. Through repeated practice, we become secure with insecurity, certain with uncertainty, comfortable with discomfort. Through staying with one method, one teacher, or one practice, and increasing the number of things we do have control over, we increase our threshold for staying with all the things we have no control over.

Over time, this open mind becomes our predominant experience so that we feel an inner stillness even in the midst of activity. How refreshing it becomes not to know exactly what is around the next corner! How enlivening to have the next vista hidden so it is a surprise to see an opening on the horizon or a dark tunnel we hadn't expected! Our faith turns from a naive one that is dependent on outcome to a mature confidence in our inseparable connection with the stream of life. Through bringing our attention back to center, we discover inside an unconditional presence waiting for our own self-recognition.

Chapter 13

The Seasons of Practice

A man went to a tailor in Pennsylvania and tried on a suit. As he stood before the mirror, he noticed the vest was a little uneven at the bottom. "Oh," said the tailor, "don't worry about that. Just hold the shorter end down with your right hand, and no one will ever notice." When the customer proceeded to do this, he noticed that the lapel of the jacket curled up instead of lying flat. "Oh, that?" said the tailor. "That's nothing. Just turn your head a little and hold it down with your chin." The customer complied, and as he did, he noticed that the inseam of the pants was a little short and he felt that the rise was a bit too tight. "Oh, don't worry about that," said the tailor. "Just pull the inseam down with your left hand, and everything will be perfect." The customer agreed and purchased the suit.

The next day he wore his new suit with all the accompanying hand and chin "alterations." As he limped through the park with his chin holding down his lapel, one hand tugging at the vest, the other hand grasping his crotch, two old men stopped playing checkers to watch him stagger by. "George, oh, my God!" said the first man. "Look at that poor crippled man!"

The second man reflected for a moment, then murmured, "Yes, George, indeed he has been terribly crippled, but I wonder, where did he get such a nice suit?"[1]

Whether we are just beginning a Yoga practice or have had an established practice for many years, the form and content of our practice needs to reflect where we are in our lives. If we hold to an immutable ideal of what a Yoga practice should be and an equally unchanging idea of who we think we ought to be, our time on the mat will become a rote exercise in recapitulating who we were or propagating who we might be. If we do not trust who we are in the present, we will forever create a practice for someone who does not exist. We may end up like our friend in the ill-fitting suit, contorting ourselves to fit into a practice that wasn't made for us. Like a suit we once wore in our twenties, it may not fit us in our fifties. Maybe it doesn't button anymore and we need to find a practice that "suits" us as we are now.

Throughout our lives, we cycle through times of expansion, times of contraction, and times of being suspended in a pause or plateau where we are assimilating and integrating our experience. These rhythmic changes are as natural to us as is our breath. As the internal metronome of rhythm, our breath mirrors this life process of taking in and absorbing, letting go and relinquishing, and resting in the moments in between. When we suppress any one of these rhythms in our Yoga practice, our time on the mat will serve to freeze our way of being rather than afford us a way of adapting and changing in response to our deepest needs.

Just as there are cycles to practice, there are also seasons to practice. More important than the actual form and content of our practice is our intention that our practice move us toward a place of wholeness. There are useful guidelines, however, for adapting Yoga practice to our age and life circumstance. For simplicity's sake I have divided these guidelines into four representative phases of life, although none can be definitive if we are truly adapting to changing circumstances. Let's look at the hallmarks of each of these periods of practice.

In our youth and twenties there is a natural proclivity toward more rigorous physical practices such as the practice of *asanas* or Yoga postures, and particularly styles of practice that build strength and stamina. Youth brings with it a wonderful exuberant energy that revels in that which is spontaneous, challenging, and fun. While there are always exceptions to the rule, generally this is not a time of life when we are drawn to do prolonged meditation or self-reflective practices. That said, some introduction to and familiarity with self-reflective practices can help to steady us in this often chaotic and confusing period. Our twenties are normally a time of taking in new ideas and techniques, and experimenting with methods of practice. The skills and habits we cultivate during this time may determine how well prepared we are for the demands and responsibilities of our thirties and forties. Thus this is a stage of life in which the teacher, teachings, and guided practice are essential. Since we don't yet have enough knowledge or experience to guide our own practice, this is a period when having a mentor is extremely important, especially the consistent mentoring of a key teacher. It is also a time when the mentor should be encouraging a faith and trust in our own inner guide so that we are actively building the skills needed for independence.

During the thirties we move into assuming greater responsibilities. With the trend in Western countries toward having children at a later stage in life, this is a time when many people enter into marriages and form families, the time traditionally known in India as the householder stage of life. This is also a period when the demands of building a successful career may be preeminent and the newfound responsibilities of supporting a family daunting. Although people in their thirties also tend toward more rigorous physical practices of Yoga, they are also beginning to be interested in regulating this energy more evenly. This is a stage of life when the practice of *pranayama* and breathing inquiries can help to balance and calm as well as restore energy levels when the demands of life threaten to undermine our health. There is a natural and necessary shift from the egocentrism of youth to a nascent awareness of others and our responsibilities and duties in relation to spouse, family, friends, and community. The thirties are characterized by a sifting process whereby we seek to find our own identity, often in the throes of strong emotional and familial pulls and urges. While this tends to be a period when there is the least amount of time for practices such as meditation, a daily period for self-reflection, however brief, can act as a touchstone to keep our feet on the ground.

As we enter our forties and fifties, there is a noticeable change in energy levels. I do not want to portray this period as a time of depressing decline, for it is more often a time of burgeoning harvest, but there is no mistaking the telltale signs of aging. We may feel stiffer when we get out of bed, find creaks and groans where there were none before, and notice that we cannot get away with the late nights of our youth without feeling the consequences the next day. If we are women, we may be entering menopause and going through major life changes as our children leave home.

This is a period of life when the focus in Yoga practice needs to shift from the mechanics of practice to the subtler underlying energetics of practice. Certainly, it will be important to maintain flexibility, joint mobility, and spinal health through careful *asana* practice, but this is a time when an obsessive focus on repetition, especially of very advanced postures, will have diminishing returns. The practice of *pranayama* or meditation or any other energetic practice that builds and retains *prana* in the body (such as tai chi, qi gong, mudras, or chanting) will give us more returns for our investment. Additionally, it can be very helpful to include the practice of restorative postures such as *Viparita Karani* (Supported Shoulderstand)[2] as a part of daily practice or as a completely separate weekly session devoted to recharging our batteries. More important, through these subtler practices we begin to realize the deeper significance of Yoga practice as the body becomes more sensitive in its role as a vehicle for perception. In keeping with this shift, the mind has begun to turn naturally and more willingly to the practice of meditation. As we care for parents and grandparents who may now be experiencing illness, we become aware that our own lives are finite. This is certainly a time when we will be reassessing our values and priorities to determine how best to invest our time and energy in the future left to us.

For some the midlife years will also awaken a call to prayer, devotional chanting, study of sacred texts and scriptures, or selfless service. If our call to the inner mindfulness practices is strong, we may feel an increased need for solitude, reflection, and periods of retreat from normal everyday responsibilities. While it is just as important to maintain our physical vitality as at any other time of our life, there can be a tendency to try to disprove our aging by clinging to practices that are no longer terribly relevant or even meaningful to us. As a teacher, I have encountered untold students in this age bracket who continue to hammer their way through practices more suited to a twenty-year-old in the belief that to change their practice is to somehow acquiesce to decrepitude or complacency. Frequently they are sustaining unnecessary injuries and feeling exhausted instead of invigorated as a result of these misdirected efforts. And, tellingly, they speak of a frustration and sense of failure when they cannot fit into the mold they have set for themselves.

This attempt to maintain a former definition of self can be unconsciously motivated by a fear of the needs and urgings of the present self and the deeper unfolding of awareness. The natural inclination to go inward and investigate the realm of the unknown requires a jettisoning of old identities, which can leave us feeling naked and vulnerable. At this time more than any other, the comfort of staying in the familiar setting of old practices can be overwhelming. In Western cultures, where aging, especially for women, is something to be fought, denied, and seen as a source of shame, there can be a tendency to turn back to more outer-directed practices just when the psyche is calling inward. We may keep ourselves busy in our Yoga practice just when we are really desiring a greater intimacy with internal silence and stillness. This can be a time when practicing with others and finding the support of other like-minded souls by attending classes and retreats can build a trust in ourselves and in the process of this inner unfolding.

My own experience with this transition during the forties is that the deeper mindfulness practices and the subtler energetic work of *pranayama* produces an immense physical vitality. For instance, if you are accustomed to practicing one to one and a half hours of *asana* and ten minutes of meditation each day, this may be a time to increase your time in meditation to thirty or forty minutes and reduce the practice of *asana*. Consistent meditation practice will address the underlying causes of tension so that you will need fewer practices that release tension. Instead of putting the same fire out each morning, you will learn how not to light the fire in the first place. Additionally, I have observed many practitioners who over years of unbalanced focus on extreme *asana* practice have aged prematurely so that at forty they might be mistaken for a sixty-year-old, and an unhealthy sixty-year-old at that. When *asana* practice is done to this extreme it can exacerbate the *vata* tendencies in the body, causing premature drying, brittleness, disorders of the nervous system, and emaciation.[3] This is certainly not the desired outcome of any Yoga practice.

As we move into our sixties and onward, the body becomes undeniably more delicate and frail, just as our hearts and minds become strengthened through the wisdom that comes with life experience and years of spiritual practice. Certainly this is a time when many people are undergoing the transition from active business life to retirement. Once a given, the very idea of retirement, however, has been called into question, as many are choosing to continue working and sharing their knowledge and experience well into their seventies and eighties. This is a time when many people feel compelled to simplify their lives and use their available energy only on those pursuits that are deeply satisfying. We may feel called to give back to others what we have learned and to share the benefit of our life experience by becoming a mentor for younger and less-experienced people.

This stage of life can be one of polarization for many, as what we have or have not cultivated within ourselves bears fruit. If throughout our early years we have not looked at what is enduring within ourselves, our identity may solidify and we may hold to that identity as

our only security. This can take the form of a growing need to barricade and isolate ourselves from any risk, even if this is only opening
to a new friendship. Many people begin a spiritual practice at this late
stage of life, compelled by the depression and meaninglessness they
feel as well as their fear of being alone and of dying. In working with
older students who have begun their practice late in life, I frequently
see a deep grieving process that occurs as people look back at their
lives and regret the risks that were not taken and the life that was un-
lived. If, through compassionate support, they have the courage to
work through this, they can receive a new lease on life.

I remember one very special student, Lena, who came to me in her
late sixties for intensive teacher training study. It became clear over the
passing days that Lena had a great fear of letting go. When she tried
to teach others, her instructions had a dry, feelingless quality that gave
all the details but communicated none of the texture or pleasure of
the movement. Her fear of allowing any spontaneity was so great that
the first day we practiced fluidic movement she fled the room in a
panic. The second day she stood stiffly in the corner watching. One
morning she came early to tell me that she was feeling deeply disturbed by what she was uncovering in herself. "In my entire life," she
related, starting to tremble, "I have never let myself have fun." Gradually, as the days went by, she began to join in, and with some playful
encouragement from her fellow students began to let down her guard.
The year following this training, Lena wrote to say she was undergoing therapy for severe depression. I was very concerned for her during
this time and eager to see her again. Little by little, Lena began to find
that inner spark, and when I bumped into her at a conference a year
later I was astounded by her transformation. She carried herself with
a new buoyancy and lightness, her voice was expressive and resonant,
and she took obvious pleasure in her practice. She had become young
again.

If throughout our lives we have developed a deep intimacy with
this inner youthfulness, that is, the eternal agelessness of the soul, in
our later years this too will intensify. I have noticed that a large per-

centage of my friends are those people in their sixties and seventies who have cultivated, sometimes quite unconsciously, this lively inner attitude. Frequently I find these friends far more adventurous, honest, and less "retiring" than people in my own age bracket. They do not tend to waste time on petty things and always seem to be involved in some new project or educating themselves in some new way. To me this is proof that the soul indeed has no age and that we can grow younger toward death.

Regardless of what stage of life we're in, Yoga practice should serve to bring forth our unique skills, strengths, and talents. It should help us live with greater ease and acceptance. If we mold our practice into some idealized form based on an external standard that is irrelevant to our own destiny, our Yoga practice will only fortify a false sense of self. In this light, always consider your practice in terms of how it can balance and serve the rest of your life. The practice should serve you; you are not a servant to the practice. While it is important to adhere to the essential teachings and spirit of the Yoga tradition, as long as the details of a practice fall under the auspices of this larger umbrella of intention, creatively adapting your practice is not only permissible, it is desirable. Being creative, however, will only turn authentic Yoga practice into a Mickey Mouse rendition if it dilutes the practice or just makes it easier. We need to be careful in our creative adaptation that we don't use modifications to avoid some of the harder practices. This is akin to drastically reducing the length of the marathon so that even the most lethargic among us can say we ran the race.

Sometimes the harder practice is not what we do on our mat but what is demanded of us off the mat. The greater practice may be in giving up part of our formal practice time to devote more attention to raising our children or taking care of our elderly parents. It is a terrible thing if we see these periods of our life as somehow taking us away from our "real" practice. Sadly, we may negate the depth and beauty of such authentic practice, measuring our success against the false scale of a culture that is itself in a state of pathological disarray. Yoga practice should not conflict with our life but contribute to it.

Whatever connects us to our essence is our practice. Whatever clears our head so we can see what is important is our practice. Once we get clear that we are practicing to live, not living to practice, we can bring the concept of formal practice into perspective. If our formal practice is utterly disassociated from our everyday lives, no amount of time on the mat will bring us peace of mind.

The question of what constitutes a practice, and in particular an "advanced" practice, becomes simpler if we define *advanced* as any practice that brings us back toward our self. In this definition, what is advanced has no outward form. It cannot be measured through an ability or inability to do difficult postures or challenging breathing exercises; these are only the outer trappings. While it is possible to attain deep realizations through such practices, being able to do advanced practices is not necessarily any evidence of such realization. This is an important distinction, both when we are assessing our own practice and also when we are choosing a teacher.

Adapting practice on a day-to-day basis means recognizing the rhythmic nature of life and acknowledging that there is nothing separate from this natural rhythm that needs to be excluded or pushed away. There will be periods in our lives when we are rapidly expanding, other times when we are taking a few steps back, and long fallow periods when it may seem as if we are making no progress at all. Let your practice evolve to support these changing phases. And perhaps the most difficult of all are those seemingly fallow times. This is the phase least accepted and least understood in a culture that values productivity and tangible results. We may wrongly interpret this fallow time as regression, complacency, or, worse, just a waste of time. The rhythm of pausing and surrendering to life is the most daring, for here we can learn to just be. All of these rhythms can occur within one formal practice session. Indeed, they occur within one normal breath cycle. But certainly, in some periods in our lives one of these rhythms will dominate. If we insist on living in only one of these rhythms, we miss the point of practice, which is to find our natural state of being.

During times of great difficulty, I always recommend simplifying formal practice. If our job is pushing and pulling us in a thousand directions, this may be a time to do just a handful of postures and to stick to a simple routine that imprints a feeling of reliability into our nervous system. Whether we're going through a divorce or an illness or building a house, if our everyday life is hectic and erratic, this is a time to make practice a comfort rather than a challenge. Conversely, if our everyday life feels very stable and is less challenging, this may be a time to be more daring and to push our limits.

It is helpful, therefore, to review on a regular basis the structure, content, form, and intention of our practice. These variables undoubtedly will change and usually need to change as our life changes. We can assess our practice by asking only whether Yoga practice is building our integrity as a human being and helping us live as an expression of our most noble virtues. Whether our practice strengthens our ability to be present with all that we experience is the only criteria we need for what we do or don't do on the mat.

Chapter 14

Intention

Everything on the earth
in between, and above
Is arising from one effulgent source.
If my thoughts, words and deeds
reflected this complete understanding of unity,
I would be the peace I am seeking in this moment.

GAYATRI MANTRA

Translated by Donna Farhi

When we read a book, our eyes focus naturally upon the words. We see that these letters, symbols, and sentences form orderly lines across the page, and we follow the progression of these figures to take on new meaning. Yet what we rarely see is the thing that consolidates all these figures: the paper. The very thing that has allowed all these separate elements to form a unified whole is the thing that is least apparent to us. In the same way, our intention forms an invisible scaffolding that gives structure and specificity to our efforts in Yoga practice. Intention, unlike paper, has no physical shape, yet it imbues objects with meaning and gives them a purposeful direction.

In truth, it matters less what we do in practice than how we do it and why we do it. The same posture, the same sequence, the same meditation done with a different intention takes on an entirely new meaning and will have entirely different outcomes. There is an amusing story about two monks and the power of intention. Both avid smokers, one day they found themselves discussing whether it was right to smoke while praying. They decided to go to the abbot and put the question to him. The next day the one monk related that the abbot had enthusiastically endorsed his smoking habit and congratulated him on the depth of his faith, while the other had been told it was absolutely forbidden and was further chastised for desecrating the holiness of prayer.

"Well, what did you ask him?" questioned the one.

"I asked him if it was okay to pray while smoking. What did you ask?"

"I asked him if it was okay to smoke while praying."

Like the monks, we will find that our intention flavors our action. Unless we know what our intention is, we have little means of consolidating all the components of our practice and bringing them into a unified action toward our goal. Without intention, all these postures, breathing practices, meditations, and the like can become little more than ineffectual gestures. When animated by intention, however, the simplest movement, the briefest meditation, and the contents of one breath cycle are made potent.

Once while in an *asana* class, I was practicing in between two men: one a friend, Richard, whose practice I deeply admired, and a newcomer, David, I'd only just met. It was an advanced class, and we were learning to do arm balance in the middle of the room. Richard would quietly place his hands on the floor, focus his gaze, throw one leg up—and fall. On falling, he would start again, pausing to consider his next attempt and every so often striking a poised balance. It was a beautiful thing to watch, this graceful response to success or failure. David, on the other hand, looked as if he might have a stroke. With each attempt, he would curse under his breath, until his face was beet red and his breathing ragged. It became very uncomfortable to be next to this barrage of curses, so vehement were his venting and strutting about. Standing between these two men felt like standing between an angel and a devil: the same posture, the same challenge, two very different intentions—and results. After class Richard and I shared a ride home with David, who continued his "practice" by berating and shouting abuse at other drivers. So unpleasant was it in the car that we asked to be let off miles from our destination. This experience clarified for me how easy it is to take any practice and twist it though our intention. Both men were taking a Yoga class, but only one was practicing Yoga.

In chapter I, "We Begin Here," we took a brief look at the primary intention of Yoga practice: to reveal the true nature of the self and to live as that true nature. This true nature is expressed through the ten qualities of the ethical precepts, the *yamas* and *niyamas*. When we have a passionate aspiration to live as our true self and as an expression of these qualities of goodness, this intention infuses everything we do in practice and determines the inner result regardless of the objective outcome. For instance, we may be moving forward into a Yoga posture, meeting the edge of resistance and experiencing the discomfort of that resistance. Without a larger purpose, we are just stretching our hamstrings. But in the context of the eight limbs of Ashtanga Yoga, this simple action can serve the purpose of steadying the mind (*dharana*, the seventh limb) and developing acceptance for where we are (*santosha*, one of the ethical precepts, the first two limbs of the *yamas* and *niyamas*). We can be testing our honesty (*satya*): Are we willing to work with clear alignment and integrity even if it takes a little longer, or do we just want to get our head down on our leg so we can look good? We can be noticing all the thoughts and distractions that percolate up as we're holding the posture and patiently bring the mind back to our breath and the immediate content of the moment (*pratyahara*, the fifth limb). Or we can just stretch our hamstrings. There's nothing wrong, of course, with just stretching our hamstrings, but if we are really interested in practicing Yoga, we can give our actions an umbrella of intention and achieve so much more with the same basic materials.

Whether we've been practicing for two weeks or twenty years, we can remind ourselves of the larger purpose of Yoga right at the beginning of every practice. As we light a stick of incense, we can consciously express a desire to illuminate the path to our center. We can say a brief prayer, such as the Gayatri Mantra quoted at the beginning of this chapter, to ground our intention, or we can sit in silence for a few moments. Our intention doesn't have to be grandiose, but it does need to be sincere. We may have a desire to release pent-up anxiety and to feel more relaxed in life. Maybe we've got back pain and we'd like to heal our injury, or we've become overweight and we've made a commitment to become healthier. We might want to clear our mind so we can move into the day without yesterday's baggage weighing us down. I cannot stress enough the importance of setting an intention at the beginning of practice, for this sets the stage for all that will follow. When we set the table for honored guests, we wipe the table clean, remove clutter, and arrange the mats, plates, cutlery, and glasses in a way that is pleasant to the eye. We light the candles, and when our friends arrive a mood has been created that influences what may happen in our coming together. How different our friends would feel if they sat down to a table covered in crumbs, old newspapers strewn in disarray, and a heap of knives and forks! This too sets a stage for the tone of our gathering. So when we begin practice with a conscious intention, we are carefully setting the stage for what is to come.

In the middle of our practice, we can pause frequently to feel the effects of our practice. Is this practice moving me toward balance and ease? Is my mind state more settled, or am I becoming more agitated through my practice? As you practice you can notice your physical, mental, and emotional state and adjust what you are doing and how you are doing it to bring your actions under the auspices of your intention. For instance, when in meditation you may notice that the mind is particularly jumpy and disjointed and that after many minutes the situation doesn't improve. You might choose to change the focus of the meditation or to change the practice altogether, spending time measuring the length of each inhalation and exhalation to help the mind settle. Or you're just recovering from the flu, and after a few postures you feel exhausted. Changing the practice by doing restorative postures and rejuvenating breath work may be an important way of expressing nonviolence (*ahimsa*) toward yourself.

When we're in the middle of practice, we can make note if other intentions creep in that are not in keeping with our larger purpose.

Maybe we start feeling superior because we're able to sit in meditation without moving while the poor fellow in front of us is shifting about trying to get comfortable. We can use that moment to reinforce our separateness (I wish these beginners would stay out of the serious retreats!) or reinforce our connection, remembering how it was for us when we first started. Maybe we can take that moment to generate a little goodwill—a wish that the other fellow's sitting becomes less painful soon. As we're practicing we may get caught up in the challenge of doing more and more difficult postures, gritting our teeth and hardening the mind as we do so. If we're clear about using these advanced postures to challenge the seatedness of our mind or strengthen our capacity for staying with difficulty (a form of *dhyana*, or sustained focus, the seventh limb of Yoga), such a practice may be fruitful. But it could very well be just another expression of the striving and ladder climbing we do in the rest of our life. Only we can know what our intention is. Only we can set our intention.

If we are a teacher of Yoga, we can pause frequently and assess our work in terms of its allegiance to the spirit and essence of the Yoga tradition. Are we loyal to the spirit of the teachings, or are we abusing the tradition for our own ends? The word *abuse* is derived from the Latin word *ab*, which means "a departure from" the *use* or purpose. When we're not sure of our actions, we can ask ourselves honestly whether we are departing from the larger purpose of the practice. We may be giving students practices for which they are ill prepared in order to curry favor, like a parent dispensing candy to a child. This has become a common practice that leaves students prone to serious injuries and also perpetuates their own delusions about their level of understanding. If we're a student seeking a teacher, we can be on the lookout for such behavior. Perhaps the teacher is in the habit of showing everyone all the terribly advanced postures he can do, and the class becomes about him rather than being relevant to the students who came to learn. Or the teacher may subtly and not-so-subtly be altering the content of the class to cater to those who came just to get a workout. Maybe as a teacher we get sidetracked in an effort to become popular or to get enough people in our class to make it work financially, and these concerns gradually change the focus of our teaching. It can be difficult to balance the very real challenge of making a livelihood and maintaining integrity. Yet when the teacher departs from the larger purpose, he or she abandons the real quest and thus removes the context through which we, the students, can pursue ours. Finding a teacher who holds the integrity of his or her intention can help us hold to ours.

As students, we may not have formed a clear intention at all about why we've come to practice Yoga, and this is why it is very important to find a teacher who can help us understand the deeper significance of the practice. Some of us are lucky to find teachers who, regardless of what they are teaching, manifest every aspect of Yoga practice through their presence, their bearing, and the way they relate to their students and to others. One such teacher was the late Indra Devi, a tiny parakeet of a woman with a heart as wide as the world. Indra Devi had an extraordinary life as one of the first Western women to study Yoga with some of the most revered masters of the past century. She later introduced millions of Westerners to Yoga in her groundbreaking *Yoga for Americans* in 1948. I remember Indra Devi for an appearance she made in her nineties at what was then called the Unity in Yoga conference. At the time the Yoga community was rife with dissent and political infighting. Even the title of the conference was a bit of an oxymoron, but someone had the bright idea to bring people from different traditions together and see if we couldn't just find a little unity in our Yoga after all. So there we were: a whole bunch of people who all thought they were doing Yoga the *right* way, backstabbing and gossiping and treating one another with suspicion or dismissal—and then Indra Devi walked into the room. Such was the purity of her very presence and her message of unconditional love that within minutes some of the hardest characters had tears in their eyes. Before long the place was like an Italian wedding, with people passing tissues up and down the aisles. Indra Devi didn't say anything particularly profound that day or dazzle us with her erudition or demonstrate any impressive postures or pontificate about Yoga philosophy. Through her simple words and her bearing, Indra Devi simply showed us what it meant to see everyone through eyes of compassion, and more than that, she *was* that compassion. This complete understanding pierced our hearts that day, and no one left the room unaffected. In fact, no one left the room until Indra Devi had embraced them. Waiting behind a rather pudgy man with thick glasses, I stood in awe as she took his glasses off and kissed his eyes. It didn't seem to matter to her who you were or who you took yourself to be: Indra Devi saw the only thing worth seeing: the sameness of everyone at the center. Indra Devi could have talked about cardboard boxes that day, and I am certain we would have received the same message, so strong was the power of her intention. Her intention entered the room before her, filled the room, and remained in the room long after she had left. Her intention seated itself in people's hearts and remained there long after her death as a legacy of her spiritual achievement.

Intention has a way of coloring all experience. Like Indra Devi, we can take the body of our practice and through intention make a movement in our life that is an expression of grace, beauty, and wisdom. We can be doing the simplest of *asanas* or meditations yet through our intention be expressing the highest realization.

We have looked at setting an intention at the beginning and the middle, and now we come to the end of a formal practice session. This moment is as potent as the commencement of practice. It is here that we can anchor our desire to bring the fruits of our formal practice into our everyday life. If the mind is more settled, we might have an aspiration to bring that mindfulness to our workplace. If we've finally managed to slow down, maybe we try bringing that leisurely pace into our drive to work. We might have the same guiding intention in our practice for months if not years. Or our intention may change from week to week. Whatever this heartfelt wish is, take some time to pause at the completion of your practice so that you take what you've learned on the mat into the rest of the day.

As we move into part 3 of this book, our intention will be even more crucial in carrying us across the inevitably rough waters that lay ahead. As we encounter the common roadblocks to clear seeing, we may find our deepest hopes and aspirations threatened by what can appear momentarily to be insurmountable obstacles. Our intention to stay with ourselves and to remain loyal to the practice can act as a life raft in these times of storm.

Part 3

Roadblocks and Distractions

Chapter 15

Sloth

The tragedy of life is not death; rather, it is what we allow to die within us while we live.

Norman Cousins

Call it what you like—idleness, indolence or languor, apathy, or inanimation—I know no better word than *sloth* to describe the habitual disinclination to effort that thwarts the potential of the budding spiritual seeker. The sloth is a bearlike creature given to hanging upside down and moving so slowly that algae gives its brown coat a green tinge. Of the nine obstacles to the yogic path listed in the Yoga-Sutra, four can be attributed in some way to the effects of dullness, laziness, and inertia. Sloth makes it almost impossible to establish a firm ground for practice, and even if we are able to do so, sloth may prevent us from sustaining any ground we have gained. Most of us have a sense of what's good for us. This knowledge of the medicine we need bypasses the central dilemma: How are we going to get to the medicine cabinet?

We all have days when laziness overtakes us. These momentary lulls need be no cause for concern for they are a part of the rhythm of life. When, however, inertia becomes a way of life, then we should take a good look at what is causing us to become passive spectators in our own lives. Even if we are busy, this does not necessarily mean that our actions are purposeful and that we are using our energies wisely. We may be as intransigently stuck in compulsive busyness as in inactivity. We may use our best energy for inconsequential

affairs—unnecessary shopping, trivial entertainment, and casual socializing—and leave the dregs for our marriage, our family and
friendships, our life's work, and the cultivation of our inner life. If we
define a Yoga practice as an awareness of and investment in our most
cherished values, we may be dismayed to discover how little real energy we designate to the central purpose of our life. So when I speak
of a habitual disinclination toward effort, I am speaking specifically
about purposeful effort. In what ways are we sabotaging ourselves,
and how can we extricate ourselves from the mire of self-indulgence?

All spiritual traditions have one compelling suggestion to remedy
inertia and ineffectual action. Consider in the harsh light of day that
you are going to die. One day—and no one knows whether that day
will be today, tomorrow, next year, or twenty years from now—the
little you will cease to be. If you believe that life on Earth is meant to
be a forlorn meal of dried toast and disappointment with the joy and
caviar arriving postmortem, then you need not concern yourself with
the issue of sloth. If you believe that on your deathbed you will be
most concerned about whether you made the right choice of bedroom decor, then read no farther. But if you believe that there is
something enduring within you and that the higher meaning and purpose of life is about finding a connection to your inner divinity, then
every moment of life will become precious. When you are fully cog-
nizant that at any moment your life could end, you will not wish to
waste your time on trivial pursuits or petty grievances. Every moment
will offer itself as a possible opportunity for connecting with the only
thing you can take with you when you die: your soul. The contemplation of death, therefore, is intended to foster a sense of immediacy
and to help us distinguish between what is salient to our very being
and what is not. When we can discriminate between those things that
are important and those that are not, how we use our time and energy
will reflect this understanding.

Many people come to this realization when tending someone who
has been incapacitated by illness, after witnessing the premature death
of a close friend or family member, or after a close brush with death

themselves. Such events often provide the nudge we need to assess whether we would feel complete should death come calling tomorrow. Could we say we are fulfilled? Would we feel that we are serving our purpose in life? Do we love fully, and what do we regret? If we are lucky, something like this happens to us early in our life and lights a fire behind us. We need not wait, however, for such an event to motivate us. While we are healthy and strong, we can consider the undeniable fact of our finite time on Earth. This contemplation of death, so common to all of the world's spiritual traditions (most notably Tibetan Buddhism), is not intended to be morbid or to impel action through fear or anxiety. Rather, it is intended to help generate a joyous awakening to the life that is available to us, should we choose to participate.

How we use the knowledge of death as a tool for breaking through inertia and awakening to life depends on our attitudes and beliefs. Whether you believe in an afterlife is inconsequential; the important thing is to use the contemplation of death skillfully and to your advantage. As a child I was always fascinated by the TV shows *Mission Impossible* and *Get Smart*. I was never sure which I liked better—the serious venture starting with that ominous catchphrase, "Your mission, should you choose to accept it . . ." with fatal portents at every turn, or the improbable shenanigans of Maxwell Smart, Agent 86, and his sidekick, 99, neither of whom seemed to get any closer to death than a bad cold. Who could dislike a character who on being awakened in the middle of the night by a telephone call from the chief and told "We're facing a terrible crisis: the possible destruction of the entire world!" would reply, "Well, couldn't it have waited until the morning?" I imagine that Agent 86 came all the closer to our hearts because we see in him some part of ourselves that wants to pretend that the show is never going to end and that we have lots of time to dawdle. When we're in the process of trying to find some internal motivation that can break through the inertia of sloth, I believe we need a little dose of both of these characters. We have to believe that there are serious consequences to inaction, but at the same time we need to be able to take ourselves and life lightly. Our *Mission Impossible* persona must believe that death is an imminent possibility, while our Agent 86 is well aware that it's all a bit of hoax and that while our body will die, "we" can never die. It is a precarious balance: to lean too far in one direction makes the spiritual path one of grim urgency, to lean too far in the other makes our time on Earth a pathetic charade. When we put death in our back pocket, we use the awareness of impermanence like a little burr in our pants to keep us from becoming too complacent.

Yoga is not a fear or shame-based philosophy, for fear rarely succeeds as the catalyst for change. If fear were an effective strategy for change, millions of people would have given up smoking already, since the dire health consequences of cigarettes are well known. Millions more would have extricated themselves from overstuffed couches and gone out exercising, chastely refusing calorific delights. Medical studies have shown that patients with serious heart disease rarely make lifestyle changes out of fear of death but will readily embrace radical lifestyle changes when these changes demonstrate a greater enjoyment and pleasure in life.[1] Clearly, a far greater motivator than fear is joy. And this is what Yoga practice is intended to generate.

The problem here, of course, is that the practice that can generate joy may be the very thing we are resisting. So let us come back to the question of practical significance: How do we break through this initial resistance? It is helpful to note that heaviness, lethargy, and depression are not states of being that anyone finds particularly enjoyable. This honest analysis can lead us to ask, "Is this how I want to be, and if not, what am I willing to do about it?" To break through such inertia takes a moment of acceleration: that self-generated push from behind that gets our wheels in motion. If you have been stuck for a long time, perhaps your whole life, it will be difficult to generate this acceleration by yourself. You may need a kick-start, a push, or simply a good kick in the pants. If at first you do not have your own internal motivation, then find someone who does: a teacher you can study with, a friend whose self-discipline inspires you, a colleague who has some get-up-and-go. Spend time with such people, and you will find that energy and enthusiasm are contagious. However, to become dependent on others will suppress your self-motivation. This self-motivation is the central issue that you cannot avoid. You cannot have baby-sitters and cheerleaders all your life jollying you along and dusting you off every time you fall. So begin, if you must, with the help of others, but do not take advantage of the generosity of those who help you. The energy given by a teacher, friend, or family member should be returned in kind through your own self-motivated efforts. Fortunately, once you are able to break through the initial gravity of inertia, the momentum gained by this effort tends to generate more of the same life-affirming energy. In essence, it gets easier.

Contemplating death will bring you to an honest assessment of what gives your life meaning. This will lead you to a choice: to fritter away your hours or to take charge of yourself and your life. Create an environment in which you can contemplate these issues with the fewest distractions. Ask yourself what truly generates joy and satisfaction for you. If you take this contemplation seriously, you may find yourself questioning a great many things that you previously took for granted. These are practical considerations, not abstract ones. Take into account how you spend your time, your money, and your sexual energy. Notice if you associate such a contemplation with a threat to all the things you currently enjoy and a life of vacant austerity and piousness. This association is a misinterpretation of the spiritual path as leading to an inert peacefulness rather than a *vibrant peacefulness*, which is the luminous matrix behind all creative work and play. You may even unconsciously fear that you are giving up life itself rather than renouncing what many see as nothing more than a living death. This contemplation both on death and what it means to truly live is designed to help you distinguish between short-lived pleasures and long-lasting joy.

I have found this contemplation most helpful in cutting through the negativity of inertia. For instance, for many years I found the presence of a TV in the house disturbing. My partner at the time had an almost reflexive habit of coming home from work and switching on the tube, effectively making any real intimacy impossible. I myself had fallen under the spell of watching the daily news while cooking dinner. The dominating noisiness of the TV made many of the things I liked to do, such as reading and craft work, impossible. When we separated, I was relieved to see the TV go and made a conscious decision that I would not buy another until I had investigated fully what could happen in the absence of this seductive entertainment.

At first I felt a little lost with the surprisingly large chunk of time now available and discomforted with the quiet of the evenings. I also became aware of how often I had used the TV to numb my feelings— to just veg out—and that except for the rare good program or movie, many hours of TV left me slightly depressed. The plethora of violence deeply disturbed me, and my mind would flash back through these gratuitous images for days and sometimes weeks after viewing them. In the absence of this influence, I soon found myself returning to activities that I had previously found immensely satisfying. I began to read in earnest again, and the time previously wasted in channel surfing was now put to good use tending my garden, cooking, or cultivating friendships. I observed that I was reestablishing a natural rhythm: staying up late only when I really had the energy and going to bed early when the day's activities had been trying. My thoughts and dreams became clearer, and I felt a newfound ease with quiet and solitude. Without the clattering stimulation of the TV, my senses became attuned to subtle changes in myself and my environment. I realized that the TV had been in charge of me and had been a considerable factor in my own slothfulness. Having reestablished an environment where the natural creativity of my mind could flourish, I felt able to choose when and if I was going to use the TV based on totally new criteria.

We can look at all aspects of our life and ask this same question: What generates joy, and what increases the distance between us and the experience of this joy? We may discover that much of our social and so-called leisure time does not fulfill us in any deep way. Maybe we have fallen into the habit of spending time gossiping or in empty conversation. Perhaps much of our spare time is spent in friendships we have outgrown. These contemplations are not intended to generate guilt or self-denial. Rather, they are intended to generate the conditions that can foster our inner happiness.

There is no need to interpret laziness or inertia as a sign of personal failure. In the yogic way of thinking, these states are a result of the interplay of the three *gunas,* or "qualities," of nature. Robert Svoboda, one of the foremost authorities on Ayurveda, describes these as:

Sattva, or *equilibrium,* the mind's normal state in which it discriminates accurately.

Rajas, or *motion,* a state in which excessive mental activity weakens discrimination.

Tamas, or *inertia,* a state in which insufficient mental activity weakens discrimination.[2]

The Bhagavad Gita describes *sattva* as the quality of blissfulness and says that through being in this state we become attached to happiness and wisdom. *Rajas* is characterized by motion and passion, often arising out of narcissistic desires and attachments. Through *rajas* we become bound to action. *Tamas* is characterized as a heedless and indolent state that is born of ignorance, thus binding us to delusion. It is considered that we evolve from *tamas* through *rajas* to *sattva,* but ultimately through the practice of Yoga we involute: that is, we return to the neutral place from which all these states arise. Knowing that the nature of the *gunas* is constantly changing, we cannot become bound to one or another. But certainly, if we want to be happy, sinking into the quicksand of *tamas* is not likely to bring us any new freedoms.

Krishna advises Arjuna:

Sattva predominates when rajas and tamas are transformed.

Rajas predominates when sattva is weak and tamas overcome.

Tamas prevails when rajas and sattva are dormant. (Bhagavad Gita 14.10)[3]

What is most insightful about this assessment is the understanding that inertia cannot be overcome just through effort or striving. It's not just that we don't try hard enough: it's that we don't have a very good connection to *sattva*, or happiness.

Many people write to the great silent sadhu Baba Hari Dass to ask him how they can overcome their difficulties through Yoga practice. When I have written to the lovely Babaji, I have always been impressed with his quick replies, especially given his demanding schedule at the ashram. His answers, however, are often incisive and out of the ordinary. Once a devotee sent a letter asking how he might cure his chronic depression, guilt, and a raging inferiority complex. No doubt the devotee waited eagerly to read about all the harsh new austerities he might apply to himself. For surely, hadn't Hari Dass himself taken a strict vow of silence for most of his life? Hari Dass replied, "There is no Mantra, drug, or posture that can cure it. . . . You have to break the pattern. Play physical games. Sing and dance!"[4]

When the mind is dominated by *sattva* and in a state of equilibrium, we will find ourselves naturally drawn toward the very things that generate this happiness. Foods, activities, and even people can be described in terms of the rajasic, tamasic, or the sattvic qualities they exhibit. Everything we ingest, whether it be food, environmental stimulation, or associations with others, can have a rajasic, tamasic, or sattvic effect upon us. For instance, eating a diet high in animal proteins and in fried and hot and spicy foods creates a rajasic effect, making us more aggressive, active, and volatile in character. Eating large quantities of sugar, heavy dairy products, alcohol, or fat can make us heavy, dull, and lethargic—qualities of tamasic imbalance. Spending time with ruthlessly ambitious people is likely to foster meanness and aggressiveness, while associating with humble people tends to bring out our own innate sense of fairness and generosity. What both Yoga and Ayurveda tell us is that when the mind is established in its original state of silence, we are naturally drawn to make choices that bring balance, health, and happiness into our lives. When the mind is not in this state, our discrimination will be weakened by the chaos of too much *rajas* or the dulling effects of too much *tamas*. Neither *rajas* nor *tamas* is bad in and of itself; *rajas* is necessary for bringing things to fruition, and *tamas* is necessary for bringing things to a conclusion. In fact, the perfect balance of these two states brings about the equilibrium of *sattva*.

How do we know when one of these states is dominant? When we're in a rajasic state, we know how to move but not necessarily how to stop. We know how to get a hundred things done, but we can't sit still for five minutes without tapping our fingers and crossing and un-crossing our legs. When we're in a tamasic state, we know all too well how to be still, but this stillness is more like a mire: we discover that when we want to move we're held back by three feet of stagnant mud. When we're in a sattvic state, we can easily choose to move or not to move, to start something or to stop something. We become a seesaw balanced upon its pivot, capable of going in either direction depending on what is needed. *Tamas* is not intrinsically negative: we need *tamas* to get a good night's sleep, and we need *tamas* to let go when we've made all the effort that is ours to make. *Rajas* is not intrinsically negative: we need *rajas* to get out of bed in the morning, and we need *rajas* to make an effort in the first place. But we also need to have a choice. This choice allows us to be skillful in our lives.

In contemporary society people tend to oscillate between extreme states of *rajas* and *tamas* and to seek out ever greater levels of stimulation or sedation. When we are not guided by the clarity of the sattvic mind, our choices will be dictated by cultural and societal influences, which are themselves impelled by the forcefulness of *rajas* or the passivity of *tamas* (as I discovered in my experiments with TV). When the mind is held hostage by these influences, our choices and decisions tend to move us in the direction of imbalance and we feel agitated, lost, and confused. When the mind is captivated by the polarities of *rajas* and *tamas*, it is hard to do the right thing. Through a harmonization of the three *gunas* the mind is drawn into a kind of involution in which it returns to its source. This primordial mind is the mother of the *gunas* and is vibrant and full of potential energy. The purpose of determining your personal proclivities is to learn which things are going to help you reconnect with this potent part of your mind. When you are in a state of balance, you are connected to your essence and hooked in to a larger intelligence that is guiding you to fulfill your soul's purpose and your destiny. This mind makes it easy to do the right thing.

In Yoga practice we take deliberate steps to create a situation in which the wrong thing becomes *hard to do* and the right thing becomes *easy to do.* This is rather like putting the cookies on the top shelf—just out of easy reach. Because Yoga is so effective in promoting the sattvic state, through its practice we naturally find ourselves letting go of those things that are not good for us. Anyone who has ever struggled to diet or to overcome alcoholism or drug or nicotine addiction will recognize that the most important thing that needs changing is not the habit but the state of mind that is generating the habit. Over the years I have watched many students who, as a result of regular Yoga practice, miraculously let go of addictions that had almost ruined their lives. Most did not focus at all on changing their habit; rather, they established a regular practice and the unhealthy habit simply vanished. This is a perfect example of the way in which the sattvic mind works to establish and maintain equilibrium.

From this understanding of the three states of nature, we can see that sloth falls at the far end of the continuum of *tamas.* Understanding sloth from this perspective, we can see that *rajas,* the state characterized by motion, can help balance this undermining tendency. *Any* movement, whether physical or mental, can generate the acceleration needed to throw off the heavy covers of *tamas.* When depression and gloom are prominent, movement such as walking and fun physical games, especially interactive ones like dancing or tennis, can help shake off the heaviness of *tamas.* Being in nature, especially near moving water such as a river, waterfall, or the powerful waves of the ocean, can also be an effective remedy for *tamas.* Even taking a cool shower instead of a hot bath can be helpful in moving *tamas.* A very light diet consisting of fruits, vegetables, and grains, even for a few days, can also help to dissipate lethargy. For someone who has trouble getting out of bed, a cup of coffee may be a positive tool for stirring the stagnant energies of *tamas*, at least initially. Mental and emotional stimulation of any kind, especially enlightening reading, an inspiring talk, a play or film, singing, or listening to beautiful music, are also powerful remedies. In my own Yoga practice I have an evocative collection of music, which I use to help balance my mental and physical state of being—calming or stimulating depending on where in the scale of *rajas* and *tamas* I fall. Once the mind has become centered in the state of *sattva*, I remove these external influences by returning to silence. We use all these and other devices as external aids. When these aids have served their purpose, the mind will be centered in itself and will naturally generate its own exuberance and supportive stillness.

In Yoga there are few value judgments concerning the types of practices we use to wake ourselves up. The tradition has always encouraged creativity and unconventional strategies: if you fall asleep when meditating, sit on the edge of a well. In traditional Yoga one such strategy is called *pratipaksha bhavanam*, or shifting perspectives. This term appears twice in the Yoga-Sutra (2.33 and 2.34) and basically means shifting your perspective if you are in a negative frame of mind. How do you shift perspectives? Consider the opposite of what you are currently experiencing. If you are fearful, don't spend your time ruminating about your fear; consider the opposite possibility, courage. If you are lethargic and stuck in a pessimistic frame of mind, contemplate the qualities of vitality and optimism. Once when I was overcome with a fear so great my hands had begun to tremble uncontrollably, I spoke with my teacher late at night. Instead of engaging me in a dialogue about my fear, he asked me to recall some moment in which I felt completely safe and at peace. This is *pratipaksha bhavanam:* changing the point of view. At once an image of myself as a teenager came to mind, standing in a light breeze next to an Arabian horse I had come to love and trust. I fell asleep immediately and woke feeling calm and centered once again.

When inertia and joylessness is our primary coloring, it is helpful to envisage some moment in our life when we felt infused with vitality and happiness, even if all we can conjure up is a singular instant when we were on top of the world. Perhaps there was a time when you were in love or you were doing something that you found immensely satisfying. Vividly contemplate the details of this experience: how you felt inside, how you looked, and how the world looked to you. Then, as you consider your present situation, allow a creative solution to suggest itself to you.

Yoga teaches that the way to joy is through joy. When we get a taste of this delightful state of equanimity, there is really nothing left to choose. When we are wedded to life it will seem ridiculous to use our energies for anything but strengthening that marriage. When we make a commitment to this inner relationship, life chooses us and we become instruments for fulfilling its purpose.

Chapter 16

Assumed Identity

> A man on meeting Picasso drew a photograph of his wife out of his
> pocket.
> "This is my wife," he said.
> "She's awfully small and flat," remarked Picasso.

In the parable recorded in the Ashtavakra Gita, the sage Ashtavakra
was so named because of the eight deformities of his body, acquired,
it was said, by his squirming in his mother's womb because he was
so displeased at hearing his father chant a grammatically incorrect
version of the Vedas. With a total of eight physical deformities,
Ashtavakra was undoubtedly not a pretty sight, and when he appeared
by request in King Janaka's court, all the assembled scholars and
courtiers began to laugh and jeer. Even the king could not suppress a
smile at the sight of Ashtavakra waddling into this gathering of finely
dressed people. But when Ashtavakra himself began to laugh uncontrollably, the king was perplexed. "I can understand why all the others
are laughing, but why are you laughing?" At this Ashtavakra became
serious, declaring he was laughing because of the absurdity of the king
expecting the truth from such a gathering of idiots. When the king
rose up in anger, with the scholars fully expecting a beheading,
Ashtavakra went on: "You see, all of these supposedly learned scholars have failed to see the essence of who I am under my skin. My
body may be deformed, but I am infinite and limitless."[1] At this, King
Janaka realized he was in the presence of someone with advanced spiritual knowledge and dismissed his courtiers to begin his tutelage as
Ashtavakra's disciple.

The first three verses of Patanjali's Yoga-Sutra (I.1–I.3) tell us that when we gain a grasp over the process of awareness, we too will see ourselves as we really are. Seeing this virgin nature of our being and living in that awareness is Yoga. Unfortunately, most of the time we don't see ourselves as we really are. Like King Janaka's scholars, we go on appearances, not only of others, but also of ourselves. We look in the mirror, and instead of seeing our infinite nature we see our wrinkles, our balding head, or the first telltale gray hairs. We see a physically beautiful person and feel attracted, or we see an ugly person and feel repelled.

Patanjali tells us that when the mind is still we perceive ourselves and the world as they really are. The state of mind called Yoga is often compared to a crystal or diamond so pristine that it reflects back exactly whatever is presented to it (I.41). This reflective consciousness does not add, subtract, edit, or rearrange the perception to suit its own agendas. We will be especially prone to this creative reshuffling of reality if it helps to prove that we are the sole purveyors of the truth. Or we may use this reshuffling process to procure some semblance of security, tenuous though it may be. Because most of us want to be right and want the psychological featherbed of security, reshuffling the deck we're given has been a favorite pastime since time immemorial. This explains why human communication of any kind tends to be a crapshoot in which we interact not with each other, but with each other's projections.

What eclipses this pristine perception? Most of the time we are busy participating in an extravaganza of thoughts, "one hundred flies to the square inch," as my grandfather used to say, obscuring the basic content of the moment. Our habitual mental preoccupation with these thoughts eclipses our awareness of an underlying, omnipresent stillness. If we were to boil down this dazzling array of mental entertainments, we would find that most of these thoughts arise out of unconscious assumptions. Making assumptions is such an insidious habit that it is the basis of much of our trouble in everyday life, scrambling our perceptions so that we taint our relationships and smearing our perceptual process so that we cannot recognize our own true identity.

Because of our penchant for drawing conclusions from biased suppositions and because we often suffer painful consequences for doing so, Yoga practice entails a meticulous examination of how we have come to know what we know. From what source do we glean these conclusions, opinions, and positions? The five types of thought are categorized in the Yoga-Sutra as correct understanding, misunderstanding, delusion brought about by imagination or conceptualization, sleep, and memories (I.6).

Until we carefully assess the source of our information, every time we open our eyes we're looking through a pair of inch-thick glasses, and every time we open our mouths it is like having a megaphone that distorts all that we say into gobbledygook. Our spouse says something to us, and a memory of Uncle John swatting us with a wooden spoon rears its ugly head, and suddenly we are talking to our spouse as if he is Uncle John reincarnate. Or maybe someone let us down long ago and now we assume that everyone around us is incompetent, and so we conduct all our conversations in a patronizing tone that gets on the nerves of even our most patient acquaintance. This habit of projection complicates life immeasurably, which is not the direction to go if we want to be happy.

The truly contemplative mind, on the other hand, is neutral. This neutrality does not imply dullness or inactivity but instead a kind of alert presence that is always available. This neutral mind is called the "witness." When we're witnessing from this neutral, nonpresumptive place, the "me" is absent—the me being whatever collection of things I have stockpiled to make up my identity (which itself is created through another subset of assumptions). This assumed identity consists of opinions, judgments, likes, dislikes, narcissistic imaginings, and all kinds of largely unconscious conditioning. The process we call Yoga is one of deconstruction—removing these assumed identities. More accurately, the assumed identities cease to operate. Because the "me" that is usually the culprit in creating this mess in the first place is being deconstructed through the practice of Yoga, over time the superimposed identities simply fall away of their own accord. This is always a difficult concept to explain, but in simple terms, when the "me" that was seeing the world through the eyes of defense, anger, or blame ceases to exist, the manifestation of defense, anger, or blame also ceases to exist. Then when we see, we are seeing things as they really are.

This choiceless awareness requires a radical form of honesty and acceptance: acceptance of self, acceptance of others, and acceptance of things just as they are. Choiceless awareness doesn't pick and choose, and it doesn't take a stand for or against an experience. Choiceless awareness notices what is. Underlying this acceptance is an abiding trust that things are just as they are supposed to be. In fact, things will continue to be just as they are regardless of any rejection, refusal, or rearrangement of reality on our part. When we can go quietly, we have begun, as Ashtavakra declares in the Ashtavakra Gita, to "relax into Life." This relaxing into life affords us an immediate experience of happiness and peacefulness that is not affected by life's vicissitudes.

Early in my development as a Yoga teacher and movement therapist, I had the good fortune to work with a teacher who had come from a Zen Buddhist background and had spent many years in a monastery. This influenced not only the content of his training, but also how he conducted his trainings, which were largely in silence. He encouraged us to center ourselves before working with anyone, to empty out the mind of busy thought, and to enter a "know-nothing" mind in the presence of our client. While it was important for us to have a comprehensive grasp of the human body—its anatomy, physiology, and function—this was not to be our primary modus operandi. Once in the presence of our client, we were to enter this know-nothing mind and allow the interaction to develop as a moment-to-moment process of deduction. The process of being with another person in this way was rather like giving a public talk without notes—daunting, to say the least. As you can imagine, my teacher's methodology (which some would claim was no methodology at all) was never and probably never will be wildly popular. A watertight formula gives us a nice neat container through which to catalog our experience and everyone we meet. The problem, of course, with any formula is that the formula itself is a conditioned way of thinking that prevents us from seeing from a fresh, unbiased viewpoint. And, although we tend to find comfort in categorizing others, we rail against the constraints of being likewise pigeonholed.

The tendency with learning anything (good or bad) is that once we have our collection of facts, figures, theories, and techniques, we start to see ourselves and others through this lens. We may try to fit the people we meet into the box of tricks and treatments that we have learned rather than deduce moment to moment what is actually happening and what is required of us. As the saying goes, give a carpenter a hammer, and he'll go looking for a nail.

One of the most devastating consequences of skewed perception is the longing that grows in us for someone to see us as we really are. We long to have someone, somewhere, even for a moment, really see us. When someone sees the "us" that is our essence, we say that we feel loved. My teacher taught that the primary thing to learn is how to *be* this loving, accepting presence. He often remarked that the most healing part of any therapeutic exchange was not the protocols and modalities employed but the quiet and still presence of the practitioner. Once people experience being seen, and seeing themselves clearly, the rest, as they say, is dross. In Yoga practice we learn to find this loving presence by self-witnessing. We stop holding out on ourselves in the blind hope that someone will rescue us from obscurity. As a child growing up in the era of Shirley Temple reruns, I often daydreamed of a Hollywood scout coming to my town and discovering me. This innocent reverie was my way of wishing that someone would see my starlike quality. Most of us live with some version of this desire, and unfortunately the Hollywood scout never arrives. In Yoga practice we discover that, like stars, we have an enduring nature, and as we recognize our own enduring nature we start to recognize it in others.

When this longing to be seen by another is great, we become susceptible to chronic manipulation of our image. We may continually rearrange and reinvent ourselves in the hope that this new rendition will please our audience. Instead of being present, we perform. Unfortunately, if we succeed, and someone does indeed appreciate or fall in love with this appearance, it will be just that, an appearance of who we really are. A friend once dated a woman who had such a fear of being seen without makeup in the morning that she arose at 4 A.M. and applied everything from foundation to eyeliner. On the morning of their first (and last) night together, he awoke alarmed by the masked woman lying next to him, who was clearly terrified at having the face she had applied smudged.

Our tendency, like that of the courtiers in their perceptions of Ashtavakra, is to make our secondary experience primary and our primary experience secondary. What is the primary experience? Yoga tells us that the primary experience is our very nature—an open and loving presence. When we're in this primary experience we have an unqualified intimacy with life. The primary experience is essentially neutral. The secondary experience is the story we tack on to this neutral backdrop. Our secondary experience is all that we draw from inference, assumption, conditioned memory, fantasy, projection, rational thought, and such things as the respected opinions of friends and colleagues who may have greater authority to know than we do. Not all of this is bad—we have to be able to discern and make decisions every day of our lives based on our perceptions. In Yoga we call this part of the mind the *buddhi*, or discriminative part of the intellect. Yoga does not discourage the cultivation or use of this part of the mind; in fact, clear thinking is the basis of *jnana* Yoga, where the mind is used to sift the real from the unreal. The point is that we rarely consider letting our primary experience be the basis of our process of awareness. More often than not, our secondary experience eclipses the primary. With Yoga practice we gradually learn to shift the attention to the ground, and as our powers of concentration develop we can do this without excluding or pushing away the secondary nature of an experience.

For instance, I may be in the habit of always having a predominant awareness of people's personalities, faults, foibles, annoying idiosyncratic gestures, and so on. God knows we're all masters at this! But if I want to make life a little happier for myself and those around me, it would behoove me to focus on the essential goodness within each person, my predominant awareness being that which joins rather than that which divides me from the other. When I am in the primary experience of myself as undivided consciousness, the witness cannot help but recognize this same consciousness in the other. Therefore, anything I refuse in the other I essentially refuse in myself. Certainly it would be foolish and indiscriminate not to be aware also of the secondary characteristics of this person, and I may choose as a result not to further my acquaintance. But even as I am witnessing these other things about another, it is helpful to keep the central truth of our shared divinity in my heart. From this perspective all experience is essentially neutral until we color it with our conditioning.

A friend of mine who has struggled with AIDS and often become very thin from illness appeared at a dinner party, except this time noticeably chubby. We hadn't seen each other in over a year, and he averted his gaze, clearly embarrassed. "It's the new drugs I'm on. Everyone takes one look at me and says, You're fat!" As we held each other's gaze, I assured him that this was not what I was seeing. Admittedly, I had noticed his newly rotund body but through practice had automatically shifted my attention to his nature—the same nature that had existed in a skeletal frame only a year before. For a moment we looked into each other's eyes and shared an unspoken recognition.

One of the pivotal ways that we operate out of assumptions, based as they are on appearances, is by assuming that we know the experience of someone else. When I began leading teacher-training programs it became clear early on that the issue of projection needed to be addressed before any effective interactions could take place. Without this awareness, participants tripped up over each other's projections at every turn, and not always gracefully. To address this issue we started practicing an exercise that you can do at any time in any situation. In the context of the training, one person begins moving physically from spontaneous impulse while the other simply witnesses. You can use any everyday situation as an opportunity to practice witnessing. When people first try this experiment, they are asked to relate their observations, which often sound something like this:

"You are obviously very depressed today."

"Wow! You've got a lot of angry energy, don't you?"

"I think you move beautifully."

"I can see you have a problem with your right hip. This means you must have an unresolved issue with your father."

In truth, if we are a neutral witness, none of these observations can be accurate. Any neutral witnessing that we did has been plastered over with our assumptions. To be more accurate, we would have to alter our statements to say:

"It *looks* as if you are depressed when you move."

"You *appear* to be depressed."

"I *imagined* that you were sad from the quality of your movement."

(Usually the most accurate:) *"I felt* a sadness in myself when I watched you move."

This is not just picky semantics. Notice that in all these statements the person witnessing is owning his or her observations and not projecting a conclusive statement. The witness also recognizes that much of what he or she is observing may be imagined, so leaving the observation open means remaining open to verification. What people find when they shift from projecting to neutral reporting is that the recipient of their communications gets a lot less defensive. Additionally, because the witness has expressed a relatively neutral observation, the field is wide open for the other person to clarify what his or her experience actually is. This reciprocal process has the advantage of helping us clean up our process of perception. This may sound terribly fundamental, but if we were to analyze our thoughts and communications throughout the course of an average day, we might be surprised at how often we operate from projection. This is what is termed false understanding.

The degree to which these projections and assumed identities affect our everyday experience can cause confusion at best and at worst be crippling. Late one night I received a phone call from a woman who introduced herself as Myra, and clearly she knew me and assumed that I knew her. Much to my embarrassment, I could not hide the fact that I hadn't a clue who I was talking to, so finally, after many minutes, I reluctantly admitted she needed to tell me more about herself. "Myra Simons! Don't you remember? From high school!" Still racking my memory at high speed (for I really didn't want to offend her), I began to get a vague picture of a red-headed school acquaintance. I reluctantly agreed to meet a few weeks later in my home.

What was most extraordinary about this meeting with Myra was that her memories of me did not in any way match my own memories of that period. Being a foreign student and often the brunt of racial taunts and other abrasive treatment, I perceived that I was generally despised by the majority of the students. Labeled the "brain box," I was a sad, forlorn, and unpopular girl. But Myra recalled me as being very well liked and regarded. This left me dumbstruck because so many of the following years were colored by this assumption that people didn't like me. It was not that Myra's observations were true and mine were false, just that there was clearly another picture here that I hadn't considered. I had some good reasons to believe I was disliked, given the "Bloody Yank!" taunts and other not-so-savory interactions with classmates ranging from comments about my height to the peculiarity of my surname. But I had taken these specific incidents and generalized them to *all* my experiences, not just in high school but for over twenty years! This realization left me unhinged for many weeks—and humbled. In how many other ways did this unconscious assumption rule my thoughts, perceptions, and interactions?

Although it can be helpful to identify the nature of our hallucinations and how these fancies may be coloring our experiences in painful and encumbering ways, Yoga practice is not a morbid autopsy of our personal history. Anyone who has ever done a great deal of psychotherapy that involves talking knows that there is a limit to what can be resolved through intellectual understanding. Now we know we were an abused or insecure child. Now what? Yoga asks, "What don't you know about yourself?" And what most of us don't know is that there is something fundamentally good and whole about each and every one of us. In Yoga we focus not on the obvious foreground, whether fact or imagination, but on the untouched background, and we bring this awareness, which is usually hidden and obscured, into full view. We do this simply by returning over and over again to the rudiments of our everyday experience. Our breath. Our feet on the ground. The sound of traffic. The taste of our sandwich. When we are truly paying attention to these basic, immediate experiences, we are experiencing, not the thing that happened to us three years ago, but the thing that is happening to us right now. We are experiencing, not the exhalation we had three years ago, but the exhalation happening right now. We are experiencing, not a past-tense person, but a present-tense symphony of sensation we can call "us." This present awareness is always new and speckless.

When we are not in this new and virgin present moment, our ideas about things will inevitably handicap us. Even when our immediate experience is contradicting our preconceived ideas and opinions, we may refuse to relinquish our old viewpoint. We usually feel the effects of this solidified viewpoint in our relationships with others. For instance, we may be in a relationship with someone whose viewpoint is essentially distrustful. No matter how worthy, reliable, and responsible we may be, we will be viewed from this distrusting perspective. Many of us experience the frozen nature of these old identities when we return to the family hearth and find the nifty persona we've developed as a thirty-something professional disintegrates at the sound of our father's voice. However we hold to an identity, the dogma of that set point of view will constrain our experience.

When my mother comes to visit, I am often on edge in the kitchen because our dietary preferences are, to put it mildly, divergent. So most of the time I don't tell her what ingredients I've used because it can be a source of friction. One evening as I unveiled a spectacular cheesecake adorned with tropical fruits, my mother enthusiastically asked for a second slice, gushing that the cheesecake was delicious, and might I tell her the recipe? When I revealed it was a tofu cheesecake and contained no dairy products, she quickly qualified her remarks: "Well, it's really good if you don't know it's tofu." A few days later she engaged my partner in a thirty-minute discussion, probing him on the intricacies of what could be made with tofu. Her interest seemed genuine as she egged him on with many questions about the different kinds of tofu, possible seasonings, and methods of preparation. When he had reached the end of this encyclopedic treatise on soy products, Mother blankly declared, "You know, I have no intention of eating that horrible stuff!" Truthfully, I have no investment in converting or convincing my mother that my own dietary protocol is better than hers. Indeed, I have made it a practice to graciously accept whatever she serves me when I am in her home, be it bacon for breakfast or cream puffs for dessert. Someone whose worldview is held together by an unshakable belief that the more meat you eat, the less likely you are to get cancer may feel that to enjoy the taste of tofu is to relinquish some important component of herself. We all have these strongholds in ourselves, and when we have our sticking points challenged by others, by life circumstances, or through our own self-observation, we can bet that the forces of defense and reaction will rise within us. The degree to which we are defensive and our reaction overblown is usually the degree to which this viewpoint has become enmeshed with our identity. We will then perceive this point of view as so much a part of ourselves that to change our point of view is to change who we are.

The ramifications of holding all these assumptions are usually far more serious, however, than our choice of protein. Perhaps long ago we had a bad experience with a person of a particular race or religion or gender and we have generalized this experience to all our current interactions. Even when we meet someone who is proving to be a wonderful acquaintance, potential friend, or trustworthy co-worker, we may be subtly undermining our relationship at every turn. Or much of our life has been filled with struggle, but even when there is no apparent difficulty and the sun is shining, we continue to live under a dark cloud.

Remarkable things happen when we become willing to test these suppositions, especially when our assumptions cause us to criticize, refuse, blame, or despise someone else. This testing process takes courage—the courage to see how we're holding ourselves up and the courage to find some other way of being that is free of this rigid inner scaffolding. Because this is an often painful and difficult process, few people are interested in doing this work, so when I meet someone who is, I am always impressed. One such person, a Yoga teacher named Debra, had kindly offered to meet me at the Houston airport and take me to a local hotel. After eighteen hours of travel, and sporting crutches from a badly sprained ankle, I was overjoyed to see her. Over the course of the next few days Debra graciously helped me get from place to place. One day as Debra was driving she turned to me and said, "The reason I volunteered to host you is that when I first saw you last year at another conference, I immediately disliked you. I'd never met you before, and I've never studied with you, but I thought you were really stuck up." I took a hard swallow and let her continue. "I wanted to know why I had such a strong dislike for someone I didn't know," she continued. "How am I doing so far?" I asked, and we both burst out laughing. "It's hard to admit," she replied, "but now I see it's because I really want to teach at conferences myself, and I feel I have a lot to offer and my abilities aren't being recognized and rewarded as yours are. I decided I really needed to take a good look at my reactions to you." In the days prior to this conversation Debra had asked me many questions about how to establish herself as a teacher, and I was eager to share with her and help her in whatever way I could, offering contact information of respected colleagues and centers. Her perceived enemy had become a helpful ally. Debra and I began an extended correspondence, and I was grateful to her for her honesty because it gave me a chance to look at whether I was unconsciously projecting an aloofness based on some feeling of superiority.

At this point you may be wondering how then one makes judgments and decisions. Is there any validity to intuition and gut feelings? What about all that education we've spent so much time accumulating? And what about the life experience we've accrued? All of these things are important components of discriminative awareness and should be used, but as adjuncts to our primary awareness of oneness. We can imagine the primary experience like the ground of our being: a matrix that can encompass all that we've learned and gained from our life experience. These secondary features of ourselves are like tiny bubbles that exist within our ground of being. When we open to the moment, if we're in our primary experience, what is necessary to the moment percolates up, and one or some of those little bubbles rise to the surface to serve the moment. In this way, what we've learned and collected gets used only as necessary and, interestingly, as a fresh response. It's exciting to meet a new moment with open awareness and allow that secondary knowledge to appear as a spontaneous improvisation. It is the same excitement a jazz musician feels when the music changes in strange and unexpected ways. When this dynamic ground becomes fused, however, we play out our lives as a mechanical repetition of a past self.

Living in this dynamic ground of being, we become more, not less, of who we are. We do not become watered-down versions of our former self, a bland monotone. Rather, this radical process called Yoga asks us to live without solidifying our viewpoint or fixing our point of reference. There is no experience from our past that need become a fulcrum for the one we are having now—or the experiences we have yet to have. When we can remove the masks of our own making, then the one who has been longing to be seen sees itself unbounded, just as it is.

Chapter 17

Measuring Up

The real measure of our wealth is how much we'd be worth if we lost all our money.

John Henry Jowett

It's late afternoon and one of my longtime students has come to visit. After a few minutes of chitchat, Sarah relates how inadequate she felt at the Yoga seminar she attended over the weekend. Just about everyone else could do the advanced postures, and she left feeling that her practice was inferior. I asked Sarah what her life was like before she began practicing Yoga and whether she had noticed any changes since then. After a brief pause, all kinds of insights began to pour forth as she recalled how difficult and confused so many areas of her life had been and how so many of those rough patches had been smoothed out.

Many years prior to meeting Sarah, I consulted with Ayurvedic doctor Robert Svoboda. As I began to relate the health problems I had suffered in the previous years I found myself apologizing profusely, which in retrospect was quite ridiculous given that my difficulties had arisen not out of any personal neglect but through a serious infection contracted while traveling. Finally succumbing to my embarrassment, I admitted that I feared that since I was a Yoga teacher perhaps he would view my less-than-perfect physical health as a sign of some serious fault in my practice. After a long pause Dr. Svoboda asked what *my* life had been like before I began practicing Yoga: Had I seen any improvement in my life since then? Like Sarah, I began to relate a veritable treasure trove of changes that had occurred since those early days, and as I spoke I could see the gradual yet definite movement toward equilibrium. After another long pause Dr. Svoboda looked me directly in the eye and said, "I would study with a teacher who had managed to improve her life through practicing Yoga." At that moment I realized the compassionate maturity of his insight and also the harshness of my own inner critic.

Since those two meetings I have reflected deeply on the question of how we measure success in spiritual practice—our own and others'. I've begun to question the gauges we use to draw our conclusions and how deceptive the outward indicators of so-called achievement can be. We seldom acknowledge in ourselves or recognize in others the halting and painful steps that lie behind the smallest changes. Neither do we appreciate that these incremental steps may be leading to something momentous. We may have formed the habit of dismissing these tiny improvements because we are holding some immutable image of ourselves that is no longer current or relevant. In doing so we fail to perceive that something vital has shifted. Or we hold out on ourselves and the people closest to us because these small changes don't add up to our expectations: we're waiting for the fait accompli before we're willing to break out the champagne. No matter how sincere and diligent we are in our practice, we may feel a constant anxiety that we're not measuring up and this fear pervades our everyday experience. How then do we measure these incremental movements and acknowledge them in a way that encourages us to continue?

First, we should ask ourselves how we currently assess the soundness of our practice. Many of us entered the world of Yoga through the door marked "physical." In measuring our success, we may make a direct correlation between our physical adeptness (or lack thereof) and the state of our soul. This is one of the most unfortunate associations that has arisen since the popularizing of hatha Yoga outside the context of Yoga as a complete life practice. If we measure ourselves by the back bends we can do, the arm balances we have mastered, and the flexibility of our hips, we will find ourselves cast adrift the moment we lose any of these attributes. Through injuries, aging, life changes, or simply genetic makeup, we may find that what we could do yesterday we cannot do today. Will we pronounce ourselves Yoga wanna-bes or Yoga has-beens? Or perhaps we entered the world of Yoga through the door marked "psychological" and we measure our success by how many retreats we have attended and how long we're able to sit still in meditation. Or if we entered through the door marked "devotional," we gauge our abilities by the affection that our teacher holds for us, or, if we are a teacher ourselves, we measure our worth on the finicky scale of how many students come to class. Maybe we think we're on the up-and-up because we're currently on a winning streak at work or in our relationships. All of these gauges leave us terribly vulnerable to the effects of changes that inevitably fall outside our control.

If our sense of self-worth is gauged by any of these changing variables, no matter how tenacious our practice is we will always be fraught with insecurity and haunted by the threat of failure. As Einstein contended, what can be measured doesn't always count, and what counts cannot always be measured. In the practice of Yoga we are cultivating a relationship with that which is enduring within us. The only way to measure the strength of this relationship is to ask who it is we are becoming through our practice. How strong is this relationship with our unchanging Self? Does it hold up under pressure, and do we fall apart the moment any of our expectations are dashed? To what degree are we able to live in a way that is compassionate? How do we gauge the strengthening of presence and this movement toward a greater kindness?

In the famous dialogue between Sri Krishna and Arjuna in the Bhagavad Gita, Arjuna asks Krishna how he can recognize those who are established in wisdom. How do they talk, sit, and conduct themselves? Clearly, Arjuna wishes to know by what means to perceive his own and others' spiritual mettle. Were all other verses of the Gita lost, the answer that Krishna gives in these short verses would be enough to set one straight on a path of wisdom: "They live in wisdom who see themselves in all and all in them, who have renounced every selfish desire and sense craving tormenting the heart" (2.55).[1]

Krishna expands on this theme by telling Arjuna that when one is established in the knowledge of one's own unity with the world, this will be demonstrated by a clear dispassion, or *vairagya*. *Vairagya* is one of the most significant (and perhaps the least understood) concepts in yogic philosophy, forming as it does a two-edged sword when combined with *abhyasa*, or practice. *Abhyasa* means "to abide" or "to engage in." The principle of *vairagya* is demonstrated by a steadfast awareness of one's infinite nature that is not disturbed by the polarities of success or failure, pleasure or pain. Usually when we think of dispassion we imagine a colorless person whose life is bereft of excitement. We may see such a person as coldly detached and without normal feeling. This is not the dispassion that Krishna is advocating, nor does he advise Arjuna to disengage himself from the world or his responsibilities. He is to practice this impartiality while being fully engaged in the world. He tells Arjuna that his practice *(abhyasa)* is to train his mind to be anchored in the joyous awareness of his infinite, deathless nature. If he does not discipline his mind in this way he will be continually sidetracked by running after temporary pleasures or running away from painful experiences. As long as the mind and senses are busy pushing and pulling, these conflicting movements will dissipate his energies and prevent him from living from the vibrancy of his true nature.

Vairagya is not detachment as we know it but the ability to remain steadfast in the calmness of one's center while being passionately engaged in the world. In a sense, *vairagya* is the ultimate attachment: a loyal marriage to the Self that resists all temptations. Gandhi, Rosa Parks, Martin Luther King Jr., Aung San Suu Kyi, and the great cellist Pablo Casals exemplified this balance of *abhyasa* and *vairagya*—fully engaged and passionately committed while at the same time unattached to the fruits of their labors. Martin Luther King Jr. contended that even if he were told the world would end tomorrow this would not stop him from planting a tree today. Gandhi advised that what you do may seem insignificant but it is most important that you do it. Krishna tells Arjuna that the measure of attainment in Yoga is the degree to which a person is firmly seated in this experience of joyous connection without attachment to the outcome.

Paradoxically, it is often through intense engagement and commitment to a goal, project, relationship, or vision that we come to know the meaning and necessity of impartiality. For if we are without this ability to remain steadfast in our center, our psychic stability will be fractured by the inevitable highs and lows of life. If our challenges in life are great, these very challenges may force us to cleave to this unchanging core within us. It is through cleaving to this central place of stability that we will be able to endure everything else. *Vairagya*, then, is the raft we can cling to in times of storm.

Like a baby learning to walk, we learn this skillful balance of engagement and detachment gradually. And like a toddler, we need encouragement with every faltering attempt we make to establish this inner uprightness. *Any* movement toward greater kindness and compassion is to be celebrated. *Any* skillfulness in staying calm in the heat of the moment, in remaining cheerful in adversity, and in maintaining equanimity in success or failure is to be commended. *Any* attempt to keep the heart open when we most wish to close down is a movement in the right direction, however minuscule or pathetic that movement may seem. When we momentarily lose it and become inwardly unseated, the fact that we have noticed our unseated state is only evidence that we have an already strong sense of what it means to be seated. Even when we make terrible mistakes and foolish errors that lead us well astray, the painfulness of these excursions is very likely to cement our commitment to stay true to our values thereafter.

Krishna enjoins Arjuna to measure his worth on the scale of his inner fortitude. Yet we live in a society that measures success according to how much money we earn, the kind of car we drive, the house we own, and how we look. We would be arrogant to think that we have not internalized this ruler and transposed external benchmarks into our spiritual practice. We begin to extricate ourselves from the violence of judging ourselves by these criteria by simply noticing how much weight these things hold for us. Being aware of this tendency to measure our worth on an external scale is the beginning of replacing this gauge with a more accurate quantifier of the mettle of our character, the soundness of our practice, and the path we've chosen.

We can do this in tangible ways during formal practice by paying attention to the *content* rather than the *form* of our experience. Instead of measuring success in practicing a Yoga posture by how far we go, we can ask how present we are in each moment. How aware are we of the movement of our breath, the sensations in our body, and the thoughts that pass through us? Instead of judging the correctness of a Yoga posture by how we look, we can inquire what positioning makes us feel most integrated and honors rather than injures our unique physical body. If we are ill or emotionally overwhelmed, how skillfully can we make this challenge grist for the mill? Instead of "How many hours did I spend meditating today?" we can ask, "How did I live my practice in every moment of the day?" Something is tragically missing in our spiritual practice if through our most diligent efforts we manage to become a perfect Yoga posture rather than a person.

If we contemplate our tendency to judge ourselves by external criteria, we will uncover many things, all of which ultimately lead us to realize that we lack faith in and esteem for our inner life. Somewhere inside, we fear that just being who we are isn't enough; we need some greater justification for our existence. This fear may cause us to engage in all kinds of undertakings that ultimately have little relevance or joy for us. Because we're not certain about the value of this inner life and whether our inner voice warrants a hearing, we try to cover all our bases by at least looking like we're doing well. While we're busily painting this veneer of success on the outside, we are often dying on the inside. Once a colleague I know, a person of great heart and intelligence, picked me up at the airport. He soon began to share that he was in difficult financial straits given the challenge of making a living teaching Yoga. When I exclaimed, "But you're driving a brand-new Volvo!" he divulged that it was on lease. But why would he put himself into further debt by leasing a car he clearly couldn't afford? "In Los Angeles," he related sadly, "people would have no respect for me if I drove a Honda."

I felt moved by my friend's predicament. I too had struggled to survive well beyond my first decade of teaching. I too had judged myself on the scale of how few or how many people turned up for class, oscillating between abject self-debasement and grandiose ego inflation. I well remember the first conference where I was given the honor of being one of four teachers in the world chosen to lead a special seminar. The class was packed with more students than I had ever seen in one room. At the end of the day I went back to my hotel room feeling a desperate inner sadness. I did not feel the elation I had so expected. Rather, I realized that the person teaching that class brimming with students was the same person who had taught class to a handful of people the year before: the same class, the same valuable information. Was the person I knew a year before a failure and the one before me now a success? Would the real Donna please stand up! Why had I failed to recognize her and to celebrate in her worth? I vowed that day not to measure my worth on this unreliable scale, for certainly continuing to do so would lead to an endless roller-coaster of suffering. Instead I made a commitment to do my very best (abhyasa) and then leave the outcome to God (vairagya).

In truth, in the practice of Yoga no one can lose. The only person who can lose is the one who believes that he or she is playing the game. It is rather like being at a soccer match in which the players are passionately battling it out on the field. The crowd is going wild, each side cheering for its own team. When we are too attached to the outcome, we're like players on the field, trying our hearts out and convinced that the game is everything. If we have a little more impartiality, we're like a member of the crowd, cheering for a certain outcome and exuberant in victory or crushed by defeat. But if we are the referee, we play the role of impartial witness, and though we run to and fro, observing the battle being played out, that's all we do. We observe the valiant scores, the sure defeat, the last-minute breakthroughs. We may be momentarily excited or disappointed by all this, but at the end of the day we cannot say we succeeded or failed, for we are neither a winner or a loser: we simply witnessed the game.

Through engaged practice and cultivated impartiality, we can gradually extricate ourselves from this painful tendency toward self-judgment and self-aggression. When we do touch our toes, when we finally accomplish that deep back bend, or when we add a few letters to the end of our name, anyone who has been there can tell you: nothing happens. The core of who we are is the same at the end as at the beginning. If our practice does not bring us closer to the inner recognition of who we really are, if we are no more loving and our hearts have remained closed, then no matter how far we progress in our practice, we have bypassed the only goal worth attaining: our Self.

Chapter 18

A Box of Monsters

*Things fall apart
the center cannot hold.*

W. B. Yeats

No matter how long we have been practicing Yoga, we might hold the pervasive and insidious belief that when we really, really get it we're going to feel splendid all the time. We may read about the blissful experiences described by saints and seers and keep hoping and wishing that one day, if we are truly good and persistent and manage to get all our ducks in a row, we're not only going to have one of these peak experiences, life is forever going to be one climactic moment after another. Like a TV commercial in which everyone is having a birthday, running into the arms of some Greek god on a Caribbean beach, or breaking into a blindingly white smile, when we really get it together, this is what life is going to be like. Or maybe we have an uncomfortable suspicion that we should be feeling a whole lot better than we are. We wake up in the morning and notice a boredom or perhaps a slight depression, and we clamber over our experience, convinced that we are falling terribly short of what we could and should be. This is the territory, not only of the naive beginner who has just set foot on the spiritual path, but also, in varying degrees, of someone well established in the spiritual life. So I would like to talk about this wild rumor because it has caused so many people so much discomfort and unnecessary embarrassment. Uprooting this pernicious idea can be very liberating, for as long as we are tyrannized by this ideal way of being, we will forever be judging and beating ourselves up about something that simply isn't true. More to the point, knowing that we may be functioning from this subliminal assumption and taking a good look at it is one way to prevent the self-sabotage that goes on each day on Yoga mats and meditation cushions around the world.

How does this assumption affect us when we first embark on a spiritual practice, and how does it manifest in later stages of a life practice? When we first start to practice Yoga, regardless of the techniques or tradition involved, our spiritual practice is going to open us up. And as we open up we are likely to sense, perceive, and feel things in a heightened way. This heightened awareness can be the source of great pleasure, but it can also be the source of considerable discomfort as we start to perceive things about ourselves *that were there all along.* When we open up, we not only start to see all the wonderful things about ourselves and the world (that were also there all along), we may start to see in Technicolor detail all our dirty little lies and untruths. All our petty resentments, negativities, personal foibles, and shortcomings are suddenly being projected on a huge billboard, and we're convinced everyone is in the know about it. We have just discovered that having a spiritual practice is not, as a recent ad touting meditation contends, "as easy and enjoyable as sipping a cool beer on a hot day," but more like sitting in a closet with a lunatic who is shouting through a megaphone. At first we may attribute this garbage dump of stuff we are feeling to the spiritual practice itself. We might, in fact, have felt a whole lot better about ourselves before we started opening up. We may even feel nostalgia for those days when a doughnut and a cup of coffee in the morning were all we needed to get a running start on the day. It's not that any of this stuff is new, it is just that perhaps for the first time we are noticing what we are seeing. Or as Sherlock Holmes pointed out, "I only see what you see, Doctor Watson, but I have trained myself to notice what I see."

So here we are, perhaps for the first time actually noticing what we see. To add to our predicament, our Yoga practice has heightened our sensitivity on every level. We have started to feel with our sensate bodies again and to feel from our hearts again, and we may experience these new feelings like a live wire that has suddenly been stripped of its insulation. Not only are we more open to our own feelings and emotions, we are more sensitive to everything around us. We get moved to tears when we hear a beautiful piece of music, and we are distraught when an old tree is felled. The most important thing to realize at this stage of practice is that the radical discoveries we are making through our newly honed ability to sense, see, and feel are not a sign that we are failing or that we are a failure. The best thing we can do when we are in this vulnerable process of self-revelation is to offer ourselves all the tenderness and compassion we can muster. Our greatest salvation may lie in being willing to visit, however briefly, these broken and unforgiving places within ourselves. The worst thing we can do when we encounter these places in ourselves is to give ourselves a double whammy: uncovering a soft spot and then beating ourselves over the head with a two-by-four for it.

It is helpful to realize that when we are stuck, blocked, or hurting, there is usually a very good reason. And because there is usually a good reason, we would be wise to uncover it at a pace that is in keeping with our ability to integrate what we discover. What may appear at first to be a jungle of useless weeds may be weeds that stabilize a steep slope. When we encounter these painful places in ourselves, we might view our discovery like an archaeologist wanting to understand the significance of the find while being careful not to destroy the site in the process of excavation. Or as a wonderful Jungian analyst once told me, "We have to unwrap the psyche slowly, Donna." When we have just found a box full of monsters, we may need to let the monsters out of the box one at a time lest we scare ourselves to death. Maybe we need to listen to what each of these monsters has to say. At first we might be able to take only brief peeks at this box of monsters without succumbing to terror. This is not a call to examine every facet of our personal archaeology or to become mired in it, but a suggestion that we gently let our insight unfold in a way that can be endured.

Early on in my teaching career I had less understanding of and re-spect for my students' threshold for dealing with their own particular box of monsters. Gradually I came to understand that *just coming to class* was for some people the upper limit of what they could endure. One day a student, Rachel, asked to speak with me after a session. She re-lated that because of my request not to wear baggy clothes to class (because it prevented me from seeing the body clearly), she had gone to a local department store to try on leotards. As Rachel squeezed what she described as her blubber body into one leotard after another, she became overwhelmed with shame and ended up sitting in a pile of latex sobbing her heart out. She felt revulsion toward her body and angry at herself that she had allowed herself to become overweight, even though from my viewpoint she seemed only naturally volup-tuous. She shared how much courage it had taken just to come to class because she was so embarrassed about her body. In her first ses-sions she often felt overwhelmed by the combination of feeling her physical weakness, her stiffness, her lack of coordination, and her self-hatred. Sometimes she felt deeply depressed after class, and some-times she felt proud of herself that she was making a new beginning. "But I'm not ready to wear a leotard. It's too much for me right now." I assured her that whatever made her feel most comfortable was the best attire. As months crept into years, even though Rachel's body weight did not change significantly, I noticed that she was slowly wearing more form-fitting clothes and taking pride in her appearance. For her, tackling the biggest monster of all had to do not with weight but with her relationship to her weight and herself. With time, she came to accept that her full figure was normal for her, and her new-found acceptance allowed her inner beauty to shine through. When she arrived one day in a bright turquoise top that accentuated the blueness of her eyes, I knew that the monsters that stood between Rachel and the world had been brushed aside and the real Rachel was beginning to shine through.

This interaction with Rachel, combined with many similar en-counters, underscored for me the importance of developing a calm and abiding self-acceptance that can accompany us as we cross these thresholds within ourselves. Without this willingness to be patient and to offer ourselves compassion, opening to our insight becomes a brutal and counterproductive act.

What can make this particular stage of spiritual life even more difficult is our strong identification with our box of monsters. We may in fact believe that we *are* our box of monsters and that we have a big *L* on our back for Loser. This is a perfectly reasonable assumption given how loudly and raucously our monsters may be rattling inside their cage and how much our thoughts about these monsters may occupy our head space. Who could have imagined that while innocently sitting on our meditation cushion a whole box of big, hairy, smelly, obnoxious monsters lay waiting? Who could have imagined that taking a Yoga class would bring up our feelings of self-loathing? That we have problems and terribly difficult issues is undeniable. At this stage of practice (and identifying with our box of monsters can happen at any stage of practice), our work will be to find compelling evidence that while there is indeed a box of monsters, there is something more to us than that.

How do we extricate ourselves from the hell of having a bunch of monsters stuck to us? First of all, we have to come to the place of realizing that the monsters aren't stuck to us, we are stuck to the monsters. We become stuck to them by thinking and believing that they are who we are. On this count I am with British philosopher Douglas Harding, who contends that in such times the simplest and most sensible thing to do is to "make for the Center, and the rest need not trouble you."[1] The central issue is always who we take ourselves to be. If we believe that we are our manifestations rather than that which manifests, we have effectively divested ourselves of our true identity. All of life's problems are subsidiary to our belief that we are cut off from this true identity. So when we're feeling threatened or uncomfortable, we need not complicate the matter by cycling through a hundred different strategies or madly searching for the highlighted point in one of our self-improvement books. We can make it our habit to head for center, the place that is basically the open space for every-thing else. Then we can be a transparent space for the arising and dissolving of all phenomena that come our way. So at this stage of practice we have to form a new habit of reclaiming our true identity. We stop believing that God is micromanaging the universe and that the monsters are *our* monsters sent to us as personal punishment. Gradually we stop taking all these monsters so personally. They are, in effect, temporary visitors.

If we haven't formed the habit of heading for the center, when the going gets rough we will head for the thing within ourselves that ap-pears the most concrete. Unfortunately, the thing that feels most concrete is often our deep place of holding and our scars. We are "survivors" of breast cancer, we are "victims" of sexual abuse, we are back pain "sufferers," we are "divorcées." Before a class began, one of the participants, Sharon, took me aside and let me know that if I came up behind her to adjust or touch her she "was going to have a traumatic experience." I asked why she was so certain of this. She ex-plained that her sexual abuse as a child had occurred in just such a manner, and after long therapy she had decided she should never ex-pose herself to such a potentially frightening experience again. "Per-haps," I countered gently, "your experience would be different today. Maybe something has changed in you. Also, this is a different situa-tion. You are not at home in your bed at night, you are in a Yoga class surrounded by your friends, and I would never touch you inappropri-ately. What exactly is your experience right now?" She reluctantly re-lated that she was feeling just fine but quickly reverted to her position that as a "sexual abuse victim" she needed to protect herself. I agreed not to touch her physically in any way and realized it would take more than a weekend intensive for Sharon to feel safe enough to let go of this self-limiting perception.

Clearly, separating out our true Self from this box of monsters is no easy task. Ramana Maharshi had an analogy that he used repeat-edly to help his disciples understand the layers of their experience and to return their awareness to this center, which he called the Self.

It is like a cinema. The screen is always there but several types
of pictures appear on the screen and then disappear. Nothing
sticks to the screen; it remains the screen. Similarly, you remain
your own Self in all the three states [wakefulness, dream, and
deep sleep]. If you know that, the three states will not trouble
you, just as the pictures which appear on the screen do not stick
to it. On the screen you sometimes see a huge ocean with endless waves; that disappears. Another time you see fire spreading
all around; that too disappears. The screen is there on both oc-
casions. Did the screen get wet with the water or did it get
burned by the fire? Nothing affected the screen. In the same
way, the things that happen during the wakeful, dream and sleep
states do not affect you at all; you remain your own Self.[2]

Maharshi's basic question was, "Are you the screen or are you the
projection?" If you think the projection and the screen are the same
thing, it is like thinking that every time there is a horror show on TV
you're going to have to repair the television. In the relative scheme of
things we are indeed affected by horror and tragedy, and it would not
be desirable to be beyond feeling, for that is what makes us human.
What I believe Maharshi is pointing to is that while there is indeed a
drama going on, this is not the end of the story. We are human, and
we are more than human. We have a body, but we are more than a
body. We have a box of monsters, and we are more than a box of
monsters. What remains after the horror show remains undamaged.

If consciousness is not divisible and if God has not divided consciousness into millions of little bits and pieces, then there is nothing
about me that is ultimately distinct and cut off from anything else. If
I have faith in this understanding and I test this proposition through
practice and experience, I have to conclude that there can be no ownership of anything that arises in my awareness. It can be comforting
when awareness is revealing the deep undertow of the psyche and
we're experiencing distress to know that there is not a single person on
the planet who has not at some time felt exactly as we have. In this

way our so-called personal suffering can be seen as universal suffering. What has changed is our willingness to be an open space for this feeling. When we're willing to be an open space for all these passing phenomena, we practice being the world.

This making for the center gradually becomes a habit that is part and parcel of how we operate. At first we may cling to center for dear life, but over time we undoubtedly will come to the conclusion that the center is itself not solid. Open awareness, consciousness, is itself pure, transparent, and boundless. There is nothing even in center that we can cling to. Baba Hari Dass likens it to the difference between a baby monkey and a kitten. When we make for center and cling to God for all we're worth, we're like a baby monkey clinging to its mother. There's nothing wrong with this clinging. When we start to realize that center itself isn't solid and there's nothing to stand on there either, we become more like a kitten that is carried by its mother.[3] We let our faith in the unboundedness of the center carry us.

How we find evidence of this center depends on who we are and what sparks our awareness of this larger life running through everything. Some people find it through service (karma Yoga), others through devotion (bhakti Yoga), some through discriminative seeing (jnana Yoga), others through meditation (raja Yoga), and still others through the beauty of nature, which is a combination of all the other types of practice. The Yoga-Sutra does not discriminate between any of these paths but simply recommends that we use the practice that is most suited to our personality. The only ideal practice is the one that works for you.

I have a shell in my home that for me is evidence that there is indeed a God. This shell is so exquisitely shaped, so perfectly symmetrical, and so remarkably tiny—so beyond anything I could imagine creating myself—that when I doubt the existence of this center, I pick up my shell. If my house were burning down, I would rush in to grab that shell. If you are like me, you find evidence of the mysterious force behind all things through connecting with nature. My spiritual mentor spent a great deal of time driving me to remote wilderness vistas just to look out at the mountain ranges, the vast plains, and the rivers interlacing the landscape. Without saying so, he wanted me to fill myself with these impressions and to understand that my interior was a mirror of this vastness and majesty. He was not the least bit interested in my story, my past, my traumas, or my depression. These were peripheral to him, and by his unusual lack of focus upon my problems, I came to see them as ultimately peripheral to me as well. What we come to see through practice, regardless of the method, is that most everything that happens to us is peripheral to this eternal force that is running through everything.

It doesn't really matter how one finds this connection to center, but it matters terribly that we do. We might find it in the stillness of meditation, in the pregnant pause between two breaths, in the deep repose of Yoga nidra,[4] or in looking into the light shining out of our lover's eyes. However we find this sense of connectedness, it's just as important that we don't identify the object with it. That is, it is not my lover that is center but the expression of the Self through my lover. It's not my ability to do an advanced back bend that takes me to center but the movement of life through me. Otherwise we just switch from one false identity to another, like the caterpillar described in the Upanishads that "having come to the end of one blade of grass, draws itself together and reaches out for the next. . . ."[5]

Let us say that we have been practicing for a while and that our connection to this mystery is strong. We have formed a habit of being in our center and, when the going gets rough, making for center. We have started to trust that we can act from this mystery, and we're wagering all our bets on this innate inner knowing. When we're not sure about something, we head for center and act from there, even if we don't understand why. At this stage of practice we may feel that having crossed all our t's and dotted all our i's we deserve some rewards. It can thus be most distressing to discover that we can still get depressed, become ill, or feel irritated and troubled by our relationships with others. Or that anything and everything that could go wrong does go wrong. There may still be a smidgen of belief that by now we should be walking around with a beatific smile on our face and that God should be on our side. After all these years of study and practice, someone somewhere must have kept track of all the brownie points we've been accumulating. This is when we are most likely, not just to hit ourselves over the head with a two-by-four, but to stand under an avalanche of two-by-fours and tell the powers that be to let it rip.

I am always a bit suspicious of people who walk around spouting angelic proclamations about how wonderful and beautiful and full of light everything is. When I meet people like this I have an over-whelming desire to go out and buy a handgun. Such people are conspir-ators in propagating a false ideal. I'm not talking about the wonderful silence that one feels around a Tibetan monk, who really is that si-lence. I'm talking about a flamboyant, in-your-face, exhibitionist goodness that should have warning labels on it. There's something, as the proverbial saying goes, just too good to be true here.

At this stage of practice we may be attempting to balance living in the absolute sense of ourselves as unbounded with living at the same time in the relative nitty-gritty world of everyday life. It can be hum-bling to discover that all this spiritual practice doesn't necessarily mit-igate life's challenges. It may come as a shock to find out that our personality doesn't change very much through all this practice. If we started out neurotic, the traces of neurosis will still be there. If we have a tendency to be fearful, the traces of fear will still be there. When we look at this more closely, we see two different levels of un-derstanding. On a relative level, the level of everyday experience, we still feel the transitoriness of moods, of our body chemistry, of aches and pains. All this is very real. On an absolute level, these transitory experiences are peripheral to the central truth of who we really are. We may have a dual awareness of our experience and of the different levels of truth in relation to that experience. We are more than one and less than two.

Regardless of how mature we are in our spiritual understanding, at any time we can experience a descent. This going under can be without reason and thus all the more perplexing. Some people describe this as the dark night of the soul, others a crossing over, others a breakdown. In truth, when we make this descent our despair may be intensified by the realization that there is no bottom to the bottom and that we can keep going down and down and still not see the end of our own annihilation. It is not something that everyone must go through, but I speak of it here because I think this is a remarkably common experience for people who are really serious about their spiritual life. When this experience is catalyzed by illness, tragedy, or a series of traumas, it is easier to understand (although this understanding by no means mitigates the pain). Or the experience can take place when the infrastructure of our life disappears—we lose our job or our home, or the person we most trusted betrays us—and everything we've built our identity on is suddenly gone. When the experience of descent happens spontaneously, it is less readily comprehended. Regardless of how we might arrive at such an experience, if we've been practicing earnestly we may conclude that all our efforts have come to naught. We were right! We are indeed our box of monsters!

There are many spiritual stories and myths about the hero or heroine who must make this descent to realize his or her true nature. Tellingly, in these myths the descent is made not once but many times, and usually over the course of a long and tumultuous epic journey. This epic quest is often marked by battles with dragons and demons that no one else in the kingdom can tame and the perilous crossing of rivers and oceans. We need not look far in our own stable of friends to recognize someone who has visited these places. I have met many remarkable spiritual people who have intimated that life-threatening illness or extreme despair, sometimes to the point of attempted suicide, ultimately brought them to the heart of their spiritual path. Douglas Harding describes his own experience with the dark night in *Face to No-Face*:

If you think of everything negative, that was about it. I'd been talking about Seeing Who you are for years, believing in it, thinking of it, sharing it, and I felt that I was still a mess, in-

credibly inadequate. I was shocked at myself for being so unre-
generate, so short of what I was talking about. I felt that I had
lost the love and confidence of my friends for good reason, that
I wasn't somehow genuine, that my words far exceeded my performance. It wasn't that I ceased seeing who I was because I
couldn't do that, but it seemed that everything had gone wrong
in an inexplicable way and that I was abandoned by God and
man somehow. It was totally foolish because on every count I
was persuaded that this was not so, and yet it occurred. . . . It
was an accumulation of my mounting distrust of myself, and
probably necessary before I could put my trust in what was not
myself.[6]

German poet Rainer Maria Rilke describes it like this:

It is possible I am pushing through solid rock
as the ore lies alone.
I am such a long way in I can see no way through and no space.
Everything is close to my face and everything close to my face is
   stone.
I don't have much knowledge yet in grief.
So this darkness makes me feel small.
You be the master, make yourself fierce, break in
And then your great transforming will happen to me
And my great grief cry will happen to you.[7]

The experience of going under is about the need to surrender the
little identity of the self. For when we descend into those dark waters,
whoever we think we are becomes unrecognizable. Whatever we
thought we could stand on is no longer there. Our failure to find an
immutable security in this small self is a *necessary failure*. We have to fail
over and over again before we're willing to consider another angle
from which to see ourselves. When all our efforts to find certainty
through the impermanent things in life haven't worked, the only place

left to stand is in the mystery of our own creation. At first the very spaciousness of this place makes it appear to be the least substantial thing we could count on. Perhaps it is only when we have tested our footing on everything else and found nothing but instability that we can step off into this vast potential and let our life become a free fall.

Whether or not we're on a spiritual path, we might ask ourselves, What is the function of these meltdowns? I believe that the intensity of these experiences, especially when they occur well down the road of a spiritual quest, comes from our *proximity to* rather than our *distance from* our authentic self. As we get closer to the core issues, the central knot, the last frontier of our place of holding, there is more at stake. It is almost like a Geiger counter giving off stronger and stronger signals as it approaches the object it is seeking. And the most astounding surprise is that all those paper monsters that have been shouting and jeering have been hiding a veritable treasure chest of insight in the center of the cage. They are furious because of our unwillingness to go beyond the appearance of anger, rage, sadness, or self-derision to get to the treasure they've been guarding. Almost everyone has experienced that dawning moment, when having walked through a barricade of monsters and confronted the thing we most feared, we are met with an immediate sense of relief and lightness and just as quickly a sense of disbelief that we waited so long to do such a simple thing. What is more, the monsters themselves fall quiet, having finally accomplished their purpose of drawing our attention to the center.

If such experiences can be welcomed as part of one's spiritual work rather than derided and held up as proof of one's spiritual failure, a tremendous internal shift occurs. The struggle, the denigration, the self-accusation—these seem to distract us from asking more crucial questions. As long as we are in that place of struggle, refusal, and personal put-down, it's like trying to drive through thick fog. When we have the savvy to remove ourselves from that kind of participation, suddenly the picture gets clearer. If we uphold and defend an image of ourselves as having transcended these kinds of difficulties, it's a basic refusal of self. There's something terribly aggressive and unloving in that refusal, which *does more harm and is more painful than the actual content of the experience.* We can't imagine denigrating a friend in this way when she is suffering, but we seem to be experts at doing it to ourselves on a daily basis. What a pity that we perceive these descents as taking us away from ourselves, when we may be coming closer than we ever dared before to the very truths that could lighten and relieve that internal burden.

Whether we are a beginner or a strongly established Yoga practitioner, there is little variation in the experience of hitting that edge. Even in simple physical terms this is true. A beginner with the flexibility of an ironing board may bend forward twenty degrees, and there it is, the sensation that says, "That's it, I'm stuck." He feels a tightness, a constriction, and an uncomfortable resistance in that moment. The most advanced hatha yogi trying to fold forward also hits that edge, and the physical sensation is exactly the same. The beginner looks at the advanced student and believes his adept comrade is having a different and undoubtedly better experience, but in truth they are having the same experience. The only differences are the place where the experience occurs and the choice in the response. The apparent beginner can have an advanced response: listening, accepting, inquiring into the nature of this edge of resistance. The seemingly advanced practitioner can have a beginner's response: refusing, deriding, forcing, or injuring. As long as we are tyrannized by an ideal of perfection we will always be at war with ourselves.

The experience of making this descent is especially difficult for teachers and mentors and those who act as role models for others on the spiritual path. When such role models are imagined as exempt from ordinary suffering, they may bear the brunt of insensitive comments and criticism when their humanity reveals itself: "How can *you* get sick, with all that Yoga you do!" "You would think with all that spiritual practice the two of you could make your relationship work!" As one colleague who is both a Yoga teacher and clinical psychologist related, "What do you do when the breakdown van breaks down?" When a student announced that she wanted to be like me because it was absolutely clear to her that "you don't feel pain in your body any-more," I remember feeling stunned and then saddened and then on some level excommunicated from the human race. No self-disclosure or admission of years of on-again, off-again physical pain could convince her of the falseness of her projection. I concluded that her projection was her own form of spiritual insurance and that my illusory pain-free existence gave her something solid to stand on. What I have found the most heartening are those teachers who make no compunction about their difficulties or their neuroses. Having come to see that that the monsters are not who they ultimately are, they have no need to hide or play masquerade. This discretionary self-disclosure is good for both parties.

The revelation that no amount of practice can offer us any immunity from bad things happening forces us into the corner of radical self-acceptance and radical surrender. If through our practice and life experience we can empirically conclude that faith in the finite things of life is exceedingly fragile, we are then left to find a faith in the mystery of everything that is infinite, enduring, and paradoxically unknowable. When we come to this point in our practice, we realize that everything we have been building is nothing more than a house in the sky.

Chapter 19

The Riptide of Strong Emotions

The world is divided into people who think they are right.
Source unknown

In the 1980s and '90s the catchphrase seemed to be "Express yourself!" Express your anger, express your opinions, express your sadness, express your sexuality. Be honest. It seemed everyone was so busy being honest and expressing themselves that few people had friends anymore. This unadulterated maelstrom of expression didn't seem to have the intended effect; it was harsh, cutting, and for the most part self-indulgent. It was easy to dish out but hard to receive. While it might have felt exhilarating in the moment and it gave temporary respite from pent-up emotions, few relationships could survive the hurt born of ill-considered words and actions. For all the pillow pounding, foam bat fights, and group Gestalt sessions, the world did not seem to become a radically kinder place, nor did the divorce rate go down. Swami Venkatesananda, the author of *Enlightened Living: Patanjali's Vision of Oneness*, offers us a very different perspective on how to engage with our feelings and thoughts: "*Yoga* happens when there is *stilling* (in the sense of continual and vigilant watchfulness) of *the movement of thought*—without expression or suppression—in the *indivisible intelligence* in which there is no movement" (1.2).[1]

What does it mean to be "without expression or suppression"? Our notions of the rights of the individual and freedom of speech seem to negate the idea. And yet here is a teacher telling us that something very special happens when we manage to stand in the middle, neither venting nor suppressing. What might happen if we ruthlessly refused to act on our destructive emotions? And how do we do this without feeling the claustrophobia of suppression?

Unlike Western models of psychology and therapy, Yoga does not place great stakes in feelings. Because of their transitory nature, neither positive nor negative feelings can be an accurate representation of the wisdom mind. As the Dalai Lama contends,

> Disturbing emotions are not of the same nature as the mind. If they were, then whenever the mind is present, the disturbing emotions should be present as well. But this is not the case. . . . Even bad-tempered people sometimes smile and relax.[2]

This very logical idea might shock many of us who believe that we are our feelings and have a loyal allegiance to them. We say, "I am Jealous, I am Depressed, I am Fearful, I am Angry," not realizing that we fix our identity on a momentary sensation and use these feelings to justify destructive words or impetuous acts as noble. I read a story in the newspaper recently of an Indian man who beat his two daughters to death while they lay sleeping because of his rage that they were going to school. Another man, consumed by road rage, attacked a driver with a crowbar because he had inadvertently been cut off. Each day we encounter stories such as these: senseless acts of violence in which emotion has gone awry with the consequences devastating not only for the victims but for the perpetrators as well. When the anger has abated, what does a man do when he realizes he has killed his own daughters? When the dent in the car is repaired, what does a person do with a prison sentence? Whether it's rage played out behind a wheel or the missile launched between two countries, such violence is preventable. We begin to create a more peaceful world the moment we develop the tolerance to be with a feeling without having to immediately act upon it.

We begin this practice by honing our awareness so we are immediately alerted when we are in the vicinity of a dangerous emotion. Instead of allowing our emotion to go on a rampage ahead of us or secretly infiltrate our interactions, we learn to notice the first inklings of an emotion, whether it be infatuation or ill will. Through the practice of adhering to the ten ethical restraints of the *yamas* and *niyamas* (as we saw in chapter 3), and the somatic and mindfulness practices outlined in the eight-limb path of Ashtanga Yoga, we become adept at knowing our physical and mental state and we learn to contain dangerous emotions until we can act (or not act) skillfully upon them. This is the first step: knowing what we feel. *We then contain this emotion not by suppressing or trying to eliminate the feeling; we contain it by being present for an emotion without the need to do something with it.*

Yoga does not ask us to deny or ignore our feelings, which would be suppression. Through practice we come to recognize that these feelings are not the most accurate representation of our true self. We may very well be jealous, depressed, fearful, or angry (and it would be wise to notice these powerful mind states), but these feelings are not all that we are. When we are whipped up by some event or crisis, we may act on these feelings in a trigger-happy way, believing that we are acting from our authentic self.

Having feelings is perfectly normal; there is nothing we can do to eradicate them, and it is not the purpose of Yoga practice to do so. It is the nature of the heart to feel, the nature of the mind to think. Feeling and thinking are not problems. In Yoga practice we simply let them arise without getting too hostile or too friendly with these temporary visitors. We do this in such a way that *all* feelings and thoughts are welcome to visit us, no matter how unpleasant their table manners. What we practice is a certain impartiality toward these visitors: we practice not fraternizing with them so much that they take up permanent residence and start redecorating our living room with horrible wallpaper. Our visitors may be flamboyant and attractive, bearing the excitement of good news. Our visitors may be shabby and smelly, reeking of yesterday's bitterness and tomorrow's grudge. It is as unwise to be swept off one's feet by the pleasurable feeling of excitement as it is to be flattened by the unpleasant feeling of disappointment. We practice impartiality toward these transitory visitors so they remain just that—transitory. We keep the doors of our internal house open so that just as visitors can enter, they can also leave.

There is a qualitative difference between being open to feelings and indulging in them. When we are open to a feeling, we listen to the content of the feeling and see if there is a message that may be important for us. All the destructive emotions have powerful messages to teach us. Being open and listening to these messengers is different from actively encouraging the messenger to become more histrionic or more venomous. Indulgence is when we act in cahoots with our feeling and urge the feeling on. We may spur the feeling to become stronger through our indignation or self-righteousness. Or we wallow in a feeling by clinging to it long after the feeling may have evaporated of its own accord. We find that the feeling that was once a temporary visitor now greets us at breakfast, lunch, and dinner, reeling out the same old story. When we indulge, we close down around a feeling, and we may become so attached to it that we merge with the feeling. Although in the larger sense this can never be true, we may become unable to separate ourselves from our most dominant feeling. We have all been around someone like this. I once spent a day with a woman who was described as a "rage-aholic." By breakfast she had whipped up a storm in a teacup because her adult son had used the "girls'" shower. By evening she was furious over a daughter-in-law who, having been given a family heirloom carpet as a gift, placed it, clearly, in the wrong room. At bedtime she fumed in German that I was "not trained for the living room" because I had tucked my stocking feet onto the couch. It seemed that no matter what the circumstance, she translated every interaction through this seething anger. She had become an angry person rather than a person who occasionally feels anger.

Yet even the most learned and practiced among us can feel helpless when a strong emotion comes visiting. What can we do when we feel like a volcano about to erupt? The destructive emotions—anger, greed, hatred, jealousy—are characterized by a strong energy; if we act from this strong energy we will almost always regret it later. If a feeling has this surging quality it can be counterproductive to take the emotion into the contained practice of meditation. If our visitor is threatening to throw plates and break windows, far better to take such a visitor for a brisk walk. Taking that brisk walk, doing a vigorous series of challenging postures, or using that energy productively by cleaning the house or digging some hard ground in the garden gives us a chance to ventilate the feeling. We make more room around it. Most important, we let the energy dissipate without harming anyone, if not in thought, then by refraining in word and deed. If the feeling is really strong, and someone else is involved, simply leave the room or agree to discuss the matter at another time. When we're right on the cusp of downloading our vengeance or stinging cynicism onto someone else, we can ask ourselves: Is what I am about to say going to make this situation better or worse? Is what I am about to do going to make this situation better or worse?

Once the energy of a strong emotion has dissipated and become more manageable, it is then advisable to move toward stilling practices. Although holding *asanas* for longer stays can be helpful, sitting meditation is often the best and simplest way to get underneath such a feeling. When we enter a sitting meditation with a strong emotion such as anger, trying to rid ourselves of this emotion is likely to be as successful as wrestling with an alligator. Instead, begin by making a thorough scan of your body, sensing from top to toe where there is tension. Perhaps your particular brand of anger comes with a tight jaw, a constricted chest, or a pain in the neck. Notice where you are holding on. Now, without being aggressive (I'm going to get rid of this feeling for once and for all!) and without bargaining (okay, if I relax, then you better go away), focus on breathing deep into the center of the tension, imagining your breath like a plow turning over the soil of your tissue: loosening and aerating the ground. If you get caught up in the story that accompanies the feeling, as often as you catch yourself in discursive thought, gently bring yourself back to an awareness of your breath without being punitive or chastising. This stage of practice can be as infuriating as baby-sitting a naughty child that jumps all over the furniture and refuses to go to bed, yelling, "Anger, anger, anger." Sometimes it can take days, weeks, or months before this obnoxious child is pacified. If we display enough disinterest and detachment (especially to the self-justifying stories we play out), eventually the emotion will stop its dangerous rampage.

Keep returning to the sensation in the body and to the process of breathing into, around, from, and through the epicenter of the tension. If nothing happens, that's okay. Just stay with it, and even if it takes a number of days or weeks, almost always as the grosser physical tension abates, one finds something underneath. This something is often the truer feeling: underneath anger we may find a deep sadness or hurt, underneath jealousy a feeling of inadequacy or betrayal. Allow whatever happens to happen: tears, trembling, sighs, as you touch base with this deeper feeling, what I call the "generative feeling." The generative feeling is the one we often skip over, moving quickly to the defensive feelings of anger or rage because we don't want to be with our hurt or fear. This process is different from expressing, which is usually directed at something or someone. Unveiling our generative feeling builds our capacity for tenderness. We can tend our feeling rather than trying to squash it. As you find yourself moving deeper in your meditation, you may experience moments of stillness, a neutral backdrop behind all the other sensations. If there is an action to be taken, let it arise out of this neutral backdrop.

Now here comes the interesting part: acting without expressing. It is almost always harmful both to the speaker and the receiver to act when there is still a strong and destructive charge attached to a feeling. Once this charge is dissipated, we often have a clearer understanding of what is going on and whether there is any action that needs to be taken. Then we might say, without expressing it in an aggressive tone, "I felt angry and hurt when you didn't come to my graduation." If we can remove the "pressing" part of the expressing, our statement will be received quite differently than if it is perceived as an attack.

Not expressing does not exonerate us from difficult actions and difficult encounters: all of us will be called upon at some time to rise with authority and assertively meet a situation head-on. Not expressing does not mean being a namby-pamby. Not expressing means not using a destructive emotion as a weapon. I do not believe that all destructive emotions should be melted down and transformed into a monotone of soft-spoken words. If we are completely aware of what we are doing, it is possible to communicate assertively in a way that transforms our anger into positive action. When we become more skillful, we can use these strong emotions to shift a situation. As long as we are in the throes of an emotion, however, the emotion will obscure the best possible path. For instance, a number of peers recall seeing their normally placid spiritual teacher burst into a shouting rampage when a ferry skipper tried to overcharge the tour group he was leading. The teacher obviously knew that such a fiery outburst was exactly what the ferry skipper expected in such an exchange and that nothing less would be effective. Then, as soon as the ferry skipper relented, their teacher resumed his calm demeanor, smiling wryly.

We should be very clear, however, about whether we are taking action to harm another or taking an action that is generated by a desire to open up a healthy dialogue. If the purpose of our action is simply to unload our psychological poop on another, we might ask what results we expect. When we are on the cusp of speaking harshly or on the verge of accusing or exploding, we might ask ourselves how often such outbursts have helped us in the past. Exactly how many times have such interactions ended positively? Did we achieve the goal we aimed for? Or did our outburst undermine any positive outcome? If we ask ourselves these questions honestly, we will discover that very few (if any) such outbursts have ended happily for ourselves or others. This knowledge can help us to put our teeth firmly around our tongue and wait until we've cooled down enough to act more skillfully.

When we build a threshold for being with our emotions, we discover that all destructive emotions have as their ancestor ignorance. When we desist from recklessly expressing these emotions, we investigate what this ignorance is. This ignorance is rooted in failing to see how similar we all are. Usually when we feel a strong negative feeling, we distance ourselves from the person or people involved. We make an "us" and a "them." When we're brave enough to step toward rather than away from such a situation, we find the person or thing we may have hated remarkably human, remarkably like us. Like soldiers who put down their guns for a brief cease-fire, we discover that the targets of our vehemence laugh, cry, grieve, and feel just as we do. Hurting another then becomes an act of hurting ourselves. Distance demonizes, closeness humanizes. Should it surprise us, then, that throughout history governments have capitalized on this divisive human tendency with propaganda that makes the enemy out there less than human? When we don't see another as human we can do terrible things, and somehow these terrible things are justified because, after all, they were just insects or animals. Hitler exterminated millions of Jews. Note that he did not kill them, as one does humans, but "exterminated" them, as one does cockroaches. His legacy lives on today as we find new sources of evil "out there" that we must protect ourselves from.

Our willingness to get to know our own destructive emotions can help us understand how others can easily feel these things too. Anyone who has ever been pushed to the limits of their emotional threshold knows that each of us has the capacity to be a murderer, an abuser, or a thief. This is exactly why we have been given spiritual practices: to humanize our demons. We don't overcome our dark side, and it's unlikely we'll stop having emotions. Instead, we learn to welcome our demons compassionately and through welcoming them to gradually tame their dangerous nature.

When we are held sway by a destructive emotion, it's like being caught in a riptide: if we struggle with a feeling like anger, we will likely drown in it; if we let it take hold of us, we'll be swept out to sea; if we skillfully use our practice and swim at an angle to the current, we can make our way to shore.

Chapter 20

Blind Spots

There was a Sufi master who made a regular sojourn to a neighboring country to do trading, traveling with his sole companion, a donkey. At the border between the two countries, a customs official searched the master and his belongings for hidden goods. Convinced the man was hiding something, the customs official became increasingly incensed. Under the amused gaze of the Sufi, he searched and researched each saddlebag and pouch and still came up empty-handed. For years the two repeated this ritual at the border until both were old and frail. At last, in exasperation the official said, "You and I are now old, my friend, and I shall soon retire. For years I have searched you each time you have made the border crossing. We both know you have been bootlegging something! So do me a favor and tell me what it is so I can retire in peace, and I promise not to tell a soul."

With twinkling eye the Sufi master replied, "Donkeys."

Some things are so close to us we can't see them at all. We've all been there. We're driving along, and a car pulls up alongside us. Because of its very proximity we don't see it until we have to make that last-second swerve. Such is the danger of being too close to anything. This is also the nature of our own idiosyncratic blind spots: the things about ourselves we can't perceive because they've become so much a part of who we are that they unconsciously dictate the very process of perception. And this same process of perception is our means of seeing. These same blind spots seem to be all too clear to those around us, who have the benefit of the outside perspective. "He just doesn't get it," we say knowingly. "She just doesn't see herself," we note sadly.

If you look at your watch to tell the time, you automatically create just the right distance to see the dial clearly. If you move the watch closer and closer to your eyes, suddenly the dial blurs, until if you hold the watch against the bridge of your nose, the time becomes unrecognizable. In the same way, when our own weaknesses and faults become enmeshed in our personality, we can't see ourselves clearly. To see into and move beyond our blind spot, we need a necessary distance.

There is a story about a noble youth born in medieval times to the knightly caste. His mother, fearful of losing her son to the barbaric plight of the warrior, steals him away one dark night to a distant village, where he is raised in poverty, unaware of his royal inheritance. One day the now young man sees an armored figure riding through the forest on a majestic horse and is so stunned by the image that he begs his mother to tell him who this apparition might be. After much pleading the mother finally relents and, without telling her son of his true origins, concedes that the man was indeed a knight trained in the art of battle. Convinced that this is his own destiny, he tells his mother to pack his meager belongings and to make a saddle of straw and old blankets for their most valued possession: a lame old cart horse. And so the youth sets forth on his journey. But because of the horse's lameness, it lists to one side. No matter how much he urges the horse in the other direction, its painful list causes it to veer left and to circle back toward the village—and the answer to his true identity.

So it is that we list: bumping into our ineptitude, scraping up against the same old problems, and returning in an infuriatingly repetitive manner to the same stuck internal mechanism. Somewhere within us a note strikes off-pitch, discordant; no matter how symphonic the music we're playing, that off-key note sounds clearly through our best cover-up attempts. And nowhere is the discordant nature of this note brought into higher resolution than in our relationships. Regardless of how many friendships, partners, or marriages we have cycled through, we may bring a strikingly similar offering to the table. We might move from relationship to relationship, from teacher to teacher, from one method to another, or we might travel from place to place, trying to solve by geography these naggingly similar conflicts, only to discover that when we unpack, we unpack ourselves too.

How can we see our own blind spots? For the most part, we can't. But fortunately for us, the world has a way of giving us exactly the kinds of problems we need to gradually uncover our weaknesses. Like our hero's listing horse, we have just the right sort of infirmity to bring us down on our knees. Or as the mystic Meister Eckhart declares, "Whether you like it or not, whether you know it or not, secretly Nature seeks and hunts and tries to ferret out the track in which God may be found."[1] The word *problem* does not mean only an obstacle; it takes its origins from the word *proballein*, which means "to throw or lay before." What is laid before us may actually serve as an aid on the path rather than the obstacle we take it to be. A more distant relative of the word *problem* is *parabola*, which metaphorically speaks of offering an explanation to a parable: Is there a lesson to be learned through this problem? A problem seen in its neutral form is merely a question. When we take this neutral question and clothe it in rejection or self-denigration (perhaps even by calling it a problem rather than a question), we prevent ourselves from recognizing the necessity of the question.

How do we know we are in the vicinity of our blind spot? We know it when we encounter the same problem, the same predicament, the same sticky situation over and over again. It's déjà vu, and not only is the same thing happening, we choose the same reaction to our problem. And—surprise, surprise—we have the same self-justifying story. After doing this enough times, we may find that our rationalizations don't hold water anymore and that our friends seem less interested in hearing about our travails. We may even get tired of hearing ourselves tell the same sad tale. Even so, when some kind person tries to point out our blind spot, we can predict that the forces of defense and justification will rise up to protect us from seeing, well, that we've tied our own shoelaces together and we're about to stumble again.

Like the generative feeling we explored in the previous chapter, which is obscured by destructive emotions, behind our blind spot often lies a place of great tenderness, a wound that hasn't healed, an insight that evokes fear. Recently when I was visiting a very close friend, we were discussing how we had changed over the years, and to my surprise she said, "Well, Donna, you're so much less angry now." I had never thought of myself as an angry person, and at first I felt a little hurt if not startled by this summation. But as I sat with this observation, I could see that her observation rang true. What she didn't say but expressed through her long allegiance to our friendship was her understanding that my anger covered a deep well of sadness and feelings of aloneness. And like the caring friend she is, she waited for a time when I would be ready to hear about this character flaw. No doubt had my friend revealed her observation even a few years earlier, I would not have been ready to receive it. This is true for all of us: we have to be ready to see our blind spot. We have to prepare our minds and hearts for this self-revelation. And more important, we have to have cultivated a capacity for gentleness so that when that moment of insight comes we can meet ourselves with kindness. Having our blind spot shoved down our throats is likely to cause us to harden and build a stronger wall around our hurts. Like a turtle, we will retract into our shell, and the more insistent others become on changing us, the more intractable our position will become. We humans don't seem to mind it when we notice a hole in our own sock, but it's altogether a different matter when someone else points this out to us.

Throughout this book we have explored the many means of seeing ourselves clearly: aspiring to the ten virtues and testing our conditioning in the often extreme weather of our relationships. We've look at the kind of effort and the right intention that can inform that effort as well as many of the obstacles that will appear before us if we're serious about our life practice. But now we come to our blind spot: the last frontier of uncharted psychological and spiritual wilderness. If we follow the eight-limb path of Ashtanga Yoga, this will inexorably lead us to our most hidden conditioning. Our unconscious beliefs, identities, and opinion are all there in our blind spot. Even given all that we've learned through practice and experience, trail and error, in the sheltered confines of our practice room and meditation cushion, we may not be able to see our way clear through our blind spot. If we're ready, there are many things we can do to gain access to this information.

If we have a trusted and competent Yoga teacher or therapist who knows us well, one of his or her jobs will be to reveal our level of conditioning. A masterful teacher will do this in such a way that the discovery will appear our own. Like a clever husband or wife, a spiritual guide will set it up to appear that it was our idea. By creating the right situation, context, questions, and sometimes pressure, a skillful teacher will position us to see what's at the end of our nose. Such a teacher will never do this in a way that is humiliating or demeaning, for to use such tactics will only once again cause us to fortify our defenses. Sometimes a teacher will "seed" this revelation long before a student has the ability to comprehend what has been given. Years ago a beloved teacher commented to me, "You have a totally wrong self-image. You carry it with you everywhere." Twenty years ago this statement made no sense to me, for that very same false image perceived and processed the information and seemingly threw it away. Yet every so often those words would percolate up into my consciousness, and gradually I fully understood what my teacher wanted to impart. Fortunately, she was skilled enough to deliver this information without hammering me, for she knew me well enough to know that such a strategy would backfire.

A skillful teacher or guide can accelerate the process of clear perception by giving us practices and tasks that can help us unearth what we don't yet see in ourselves. Rather than stating the obvious, she or he will give us a difficult practice through which we discover the obvious. In a private meeting with the silent sadhu Baba Hari Dass, I brought him questions about how to get over a painful attachment to an unhealthy relationship. "Should I practice celibacy, Baba?" At this his eyes glittered with amusement and he began to laugh uncontrollably. When at last his laughter had abated, he wrote on his chalkboard, "You!" This seemed to bring on another fit of mirth. Seeing how clearly discomforted and confused I was, for I was barely into my twenties, he added, "Find a replacement." But just as I was about to leave, Baba Hari Dass became serious and offered, "But first, you must learn how to be friends with men." This final advice led quite naturally to a period of three years of celibacy, which were completely without conflict for me, as I did indeed learn to be friends with men.

We can also accelerate the process of perceiving clearly by asking our closest friends, our family, and those whose judgment we trust to tell us honestly what they see. This takes great courage and is not for the faint of heart. This is such an unusual request that most friends and family will honor it by being extremely reserved in their observations. We should be certain that the person we have chosen is wise. We should also be certain that we are truly ready to hear what she or he might say. A friend like this is a gift to be cherished. Such a friend is not only telling us something about ourselves that is onerous, she or he undoubtedly has had to live with and accept this very same thing about us. Our friend has lived through our depression, our self-righteous tirades, our quick anger. He or she has been there when the chips are down and we're dusting ourselves off after our last fiasco. A friend who can tell us we have spinach between our teeth is a friend who should be rewarded with our thanks rather than our defense. Whether someone tells us, or we manage to see our blind spot on our own, it's imperative to just allow ourselves to be with this revelation. We can create the necessary distance for seeing clearly by spending time with this information instead of reacting in the moment.

When I still lived in the United States I led an annual women's retreat in northern California. One participant, Kathryn, came each year, and each year she created the same painful predicament. Within a few days of the start of the retreat, all the other participants began to move away from Kathryn, taking deliberate steps to avoid her. As the leader of the group, I was very sad watching this predicable progression. Kathryn had such a strong desire and need to be included that her only way of interacting with others was to dominate: to interrupt by butting into conversations, to take center stage in class by bombarding me with questions, or when all else failed, to be passively oblivious to the needs of others. Whether stomping in her hiking boots across the dormitory floor in the early hours of the morning or turning on her hair dryer at midnight, Kathryn had a way of infuriating people. As could be predicted, retreatants began to come to me with complaints ("Does she have to bring her electric toothbrush on the morning hike?"), and when the cook threatened to quit (narrowly averted by ministrations of chamomile tea) I knew it was time to act. Taking Kathryn aside, I told her I recognized in her a good heart and a generous spirit, but sometimes I felt frightened that no matter how much I helped her in class, no matter how many questions I answered, my response would never be enough. I told her that I felt frightened by my inability to meet her needs, which seem to grow larger the more I gave. Kathryn began to relate how she didn't trust that she was going to get what she needed unless she controlled situations. I shared that many of the participants found this behavior off-putting and that her strategy was having the opposite effect of the one she intended. Obviously these were very difficult things to communicate, but to Kathryn's credit she began to approach other retreatants, asking them to be honest with her about why they didn't include her. This was something people could relate to. Her fellow yoginis began to feel a tenderness for Kathryn—the very real hurt she felt in being excluded and how much she wanted to belong. Gradually, as the retreat drew to a close, people softened toward Kathryn and invited her to join them on outings.

Telling someone about a blind spot that we perceive to be a cause of his or her suffering is tricky business. More often than not, revealing the blind spot of someone, even someone we love very much, can be a strategy for unloading our growing criticism. It would be even more foolish to engage with a person with whom we do not already have a constructive relationship. When we're not sure about the wisdom of doing so, we might ask, "Is what I am about to say likely to make a positive difference?" and "Am I the person to say this?" and "Is this the time to say it?" When all three of these factors coincide, sharing this information with a spiritual friend can be powerful and useful. Because these three factors are rarely in a neat constellation, we may have to develop some radical patience. This radical patience is one of the most arduous of all spiritual practices, yet when we develop tolerance for others we sow a seed of tolerance for our own fumblings. A Sufi friend who has since passed on held tolerance as the highest spiritual virtue, but when delivery of an unpleasant message was warranted he advised, "Always wrap your bitter message in humor first." This wrapping of the message has a way of communicating our own empathy for a foible. Wrapping a message can take the form of admitting that we too struggle with the same character fault. Instead of saying, "I wish you weren't such an angry person!" we can say, "I find it hard sometimes to control my anger too" and "I'm new at this, but I've found that when I do contain my anger it prevents a bad situation from becoming worse."

One of my long-standing students, Rebecca, has carried with her a terrible anxiety that she's not going to "get it." This anxiety reveals itself the moment she speaks, her words hurried along in a breathless flurry of urgency and self-doubt. This habit of speaking in a rush has the effect of making others around her anxious and edgy. Even at the end of a long three-hour class in which assistants have given her extra attention, or I've made her the central focus, she will stay afterward, placing herself a few inches away from my face, wanting more. More advice. More techniques. More encouragement. During one intensive I asked Rebecca to make it her practice to pause before speaking and to speak slowly enough that she could feel the natural cadence of her breath rhythm. This might sound simple, but for Rebecca this practice was akin to changing the way she walked. Rebecca needed lots of reminders, for in an instant she'd be talking a mile a minute, working herself into a fluster. This habit no doubt underscored a deep fear of letting go—a feeling that without pushing a situation from behind or pulling it from the front, Rebecca wasn't going to "get there." Without criticizing her, her fellow students gently reminded Rebecca to slow down and gave her glowing praise when she told of some insight without rushing. One day, as she once again stayed behind to ask for more help and placed herself in a demandingly close physical stance, I told Rebecca that I could not answer her questions. This surprised her, but I could sense she was ready. As gently as I could, I told Rebecca that her habit of seeking the answers to her questions was moving her further away from the very source of those answers: she could find these answers in relaxing and learning to trust her own insight. Since I had worked with Rebecca for many years, she knew that my message was not an attempt to hurt her in any way. For the next few days Rebecca was very quiet, and then in our final session she related in the closing circle what she had learned. I cannot remember exactly what Rebecca said that day, only the amazed looks of her fellow students as she spoke, perhaps for the first time, in a calm and relaxed way. When she had finished the group broke into spontaneous applause at Rebecca's breakthrough and her courage.

Revealing a blind spot prematurely can be an act of violence. Whether we are a teacher, a friend, a parent, or a spouse, balancing the *yamas* of truthfulness *(satya)* and nonviolence *(ahimsa)* can be like trying to tap-dance on greased bowling balls. Can we tell the truth in a way that isn't a deliberate attempt to inflict suffering? Can we be compassionate without avoiding the staunch task of being truthful? We should be certain, when we do speak or act, that we've contained any underlying feelings of rage or impatience so that we don't use the opportunity as an excuse to get in a few low blows at the same time. In the pressure cooker of intimate relationships this can be a challenging practice. More radical still is to accept that our spouse, friend, or student may never see his or her blind spot. For that matter, we may never see our own intransigent holding places. Trying to change ourselves and trying to change others is more often than not a covert act of self-aggression. In Yoga practice we create a context in which change can occur, a situation in which it is most likely that we can come to these places of self-revelation. Beyond this work, all we can do is let go and accept exactly where we are.

All Yoga practices lead to seeing things as they are. In Yoga we practice opening the mind, softening the heart, and in doing so we make ourselves at once invincible and vulnerable. We achieve this by relaxing the mind, releasing tension in the body, and allowing whatever is in the field of awareness to arise and to dissolve. When we notice a clinging to an experience, as is so common when we blame or when we're squarely in the middle of a difficult emotion, the practice of softening is more difficult, but it is not impossible. We can learn to bring an impartial and compassionate eye to those problems that recur again and again and ask, as Rebecca did, to see the message. Instead of running away, we can sit still, breathe, and watch. When we can admit that maybe we don't know everything yet, and maybe there are some things about ourselves we might not be able to see, we bring an attitude of humility to the practice. Together with the practice of impartiality, which gives us enough distance for things to come into focus, this humility kindles a compassion for our own blindness. When this humility is sincere, we send a clear message to the universe that we would like to see ourselves as we really are. When we begin such a friendship with our hidden faults, we will inevitably be led by the hand into the heart of the self.

Like Any Other Day

*Han Shan, that great and crazy Chinese poet a thousand years ago,
said we're all like bugs in a bowl—all day goin' around never leaving
their bowl. I say that's right every day climbing up the side, slidin' back
down over and over again. Sit in the bottom of the bowl head in your
hands—cry—moan—feel sorry for yourself. Or—look around . . .
see your fellow bugs—walk around say "how ya doin'?" Say "hey,
nice bowl."*

David Buttfeld

Does Yoga practice make life easier? Most assuredly, all that is onerous and cumbersome does not go away. Yet our once implacable desire for certainty wavers in the face of something better: living in awe,
wonder, and delight. Life does not become easier; we become easier
with life just as it is, without conclusions, fail-safe securities, or the
promise of happily-ever-after endings. If our practice fails to offer us
such sureties it is a necessary failure, for the soul does not flourish in
such conditions. It is just this openness of the body, mind, and heart
that makes available to us the largest possible life. We become less
hindered by our past and less invested in our fantasies. Instead we
begin to live with a sense of immediacy and lucidity that makes
everything we encounter—good, bad, and indifferent—illumined
through awareness.

We practice on and off our mat to enlighten our living. Nothing has
changed. Still the difficulties, the challenges, the moments of doubt, the
evening time of aloneness. Still the world with all its harsh realities,
cruel fortunes, and unequivocal demands. Still the misunderstandings,
the necessary compromises, the breakthroughs and triumphs. Still the

ups and downs. Practice cannot and does not eliminate these ex-
tremes. *What practice does do is give us direct access to an internal and ever-present
refuge of peacefulness that exists inside of and despite all polarities.* If our practice
has tethered us to life, we stop feeling so threatened by all these com-
ings and goings. We learn to thread what is burdensome next to that
which is pleasant. We thread what is painful next to what is pleasurable. We thread our foibles and strengths side by side. We thread the
seemingly incongruous nature of everyday life, full of awkward irreg-
ularity and irony, with our aspirations to clarity, calm, and order.
Threaded to everything, we can take delight in this peculiar and perplexing thing called life. We make it our task, then, to love what we
cannot possibly understand by letting the mind lie down and the wisdom of the heart take over.

Does Yoga practice change who we are? We remain exactly the
same except for one extraordinary difference. We see ourselves and
the world differently, for we see ourselves *as* the world, and in doing
so we find we have less need to barricade ourselves from a perceived
other. In dismantling these barriers of separation, we develop a fearlessness in relation to this largeness that allows us to step forward
where we once held back. We see the same things, but now we actually notice what we see. We hear the same things, but now we notice
what we hear. We feel, taste, and touch the same things but through
an intensified register.

This Yoga, this enlightened way of living, leads us to a clarity that
does not exist of itself and by itself. Gradually it occurs to us that becoming clear is imperative not only for our own well-being but for the
present and future world in which we live. We may begin practicing
Yoga because of justifiably selfish reasons, and there is nothing wrong
with such motivations if they set our feet firmly on the path. If we do
not advance beyond these initial motivations, however, the introverted
practices of Yoga will tend to cultivate a growing spiritual narcissism
that can become an obstacle to spiritual maturity.

Coming to the Buddhist Yoga ideal of the *bodhisattva,* or the spiritual practitioner who engages in the practice and attainment of clarity

for the sake of others, is rarely a commitment we make after our first Yoga class. We may come to this awareness when we feel we have a firmly established inner centeredness and a steady if not altogether accomplished grasp of our worldly affairs. Once we have established this solid foundation, a certain malaise or complacency may set in, and it is at such a time that we may begin searching for a more compelling reason to practice than reaching the thirty-minute mark in our headstand. When I began my Yoga practice at the budding age of sixteen, I was primarily interested in quenching my fear, but I was equally motivated by the possibility that I too could look like Richard Hittleman's model, Cheryl. With her long straight hair and impossibly thin frame, Cheryl looked like if she stepped out into a rainy day she would not get wet. Since I was five-foot-two, pudgy, and endowed with frantically curly hair, it was improbable that I would attain Cheryldom. But I am grateful to Cheryl for the way she motivated my early attempts at Yoga practice. I am equally grateful that not long after these first forays I met a Yoga teacher who from her first opening words clearly communicated that this practice had something more than weight loss as its end result. We need not feel apologetic for the reasons we began Yoga practice, but if we are still looking for Cheryldom or some equivalent twenty years down the track, it's time to reassess our intentions. For the inner expansion of oneself as a human being is always intimately tied to one's relationship with the world.

We serve others by living our dharma completely. The word *dharma* has many meanings. It can mean duty, but it can also speak of a soul purpose that we alone can accomplish. In the Bhagavad Gita Krishna advises Arjuna, "It is better to perform one's own duties imperfectly than to master the duties of another. By fulfilling the obligations he is born with, a person never comes to grief" (18.47).[1] We may feel that what we do is insignificant or unimportant. Perhaps we trivialize our role in raising our children, or we rail against the necessity of mundane administrative tasks even for a worthy purpose. Anticipating this rejoinder, Krishna declares:

No one should abandon duties
because he sees defects in them.
Every action, every activity, is surrounded
by defects as a fire is surrounded by smoke. (18.47)[2]

We may also feel that our dharma is a tough road to follow especially when our path leads into uncharted territory and goes against
the grain of our cultural indoctrination. The steep incline of such a
path is a mark of its authenticity, and if we can find our angle of repose here we can find it anywhere. Finding that angle of repose here
will actually mean something because this balance has been attained
in real terms, in the real world and not simply in the sequestered
comfort we find perched on our meditation cushion.

How do we know whether a path or action is our dharma? Our
dharma is almost always the option we choose last because it is the
most challenging. It is not the rose garden path with park benches
strategically placed for our convenience. Rather, it's the path that
looks like an Outward Bound course designed by someone with a
brutish sense of humor. When we first come upon our dharma it may
feel as if we're staring up at a sheer rock face and no one has bothered
to put in the handholds for us. When Arjuna trembles before the
battle that awaits him, it is not only out of fear, it is out of an implicit
knowledge that this battle is his *only* choice if he is to live his dharma.
Fortunately, living one's dharma gets easier, for the action of choosing
the road less traveled brings us up against enough lions and tigers to
cultivate fearlessness. We get better at the emotional rappel, the psychological free fall, and the tenacious reach toward our goal. We discover that living our dharma is the most creative stance to take when
we feel hopeless or filled with despair, for it helps us look for opportunities to put our strength to good uses.

This larger vision of what we can be and what this means for the
world ennobles our practice. When we have a deeply felt sense that
our life practice is important to the world, this awareness acts as a
steady impetus and provides an energy that we might not be able to

conjure just for ourselves. When our own personal dharma affects and involves others, this responsibility can goad us to do our best when we might be more inclined to take a backseat. The impetus of this intention can lighten even the most burdensome task and act to forge a path through obstacles that cannot be removed any other way. An ennobling vision takes what may seem paltry and insignificant in the context of one Yoga mat and one person and gives a larger ultimate significance to the practice. This encompassing vision helps us remove the largest and most intransigent of all obstacles in our yogic path—the belief that we stand alone outside the circle in which all humanity is gathered.

If we haven't yet come to this inclusive awareness, we can begin to seed this possibility in our daily practice. The practice of the four *brahmavihara* discussed in chapter 6 are central to breaking down the arbitrary barriers between self and other. It may be worthwhile to review them here. The four qualities of heart are:

1. Friendliness toward the joyful
2. Compassion for those who are suffering
3. Celebrating the good in others
4. Remaining impartial to the faults and imperfections of others (Yoga-Sutra 1.33)

These qualities of heart can help us make the necessary link between our personal practice and the universal application and consequence of that practice. We can also make the practice of the *yamas*, or "outer restraints," and *niyamas*, or "inner restraints," a source of deep contemplation on our thoughts, words, and actions. The practices of not-harming *(ahimsa)*, truthfulness *(satya)*, not-stealing *(asteya)*, using our energy wisely *(brahmacharya)*, and not-grasping *(aparigraha)* can help us to determine right action in the world. We can take any one of the *yamas*, as Gandhi did with his vow of nonviolence, and plumb it deeply, making it the central source of our meditation or commitment in our life. When we take the practice of even one of these precepts to heart, it will lead us into an understanding of the others. Perhaps we're interested in the precept of *aparigraha*, not-stealing or, more positively framed, the attitude of generosity. Maybe we reconsider our thinking at our workplace, looking at how much we can give our employees rather than how little. When someone rips us off or leaves us with the short end of the stick, we start to contemplate the immediate and long-term consequences that follow. Rather than practicing the *yamas* blindly, we test their soundness by looking at the depth and breadth to which they can be applied and the effect of their application on ourselves and on others, in the short term and in the long term.

These attitudes and qualities of heart as they relate to the other are prerequisites to the *niyamas*, or "inner observances," which relate to the personal self. Why? Because interacting in the world in an ethical way not only sets up the conditions to make these inner observances easier, it also dismantles the false sense of separation that keeps us from living joyously in the realization of our true nature. This true nature is exemplified by the five *niyamas*, or inner observances, of purity, contentment, burning enthusiasm, self-study, and celebration of life. We find that there is a direct relationship between honesty with others and our own contentment. When we deceive others, we live in perpetual conflict. When we're driven by greed, we find ourselves unable to feel content no matter how much we have, or we live with anxiety that what we do have will be taken away from us. If we look at the consequences of our interactions in the world, we inevitably discover that we're part of an infinitely woven web and that a pull on one strand affects all the others. Most compellingly, when we stick to these yogic principles and test the precepts over the long haul, we find that practicing them does make a difference. By refusing to perpetuate the norm, we change the norm.

This intimacy with the world may not be apparent when we are seated, apparently alone, in our practice room. With conscious effort, however, we can acquire a grasp of the larger context in which our personal practice takes place. One practice, which I call the Body of the World meditation, can be done in *Savasana*, Corpse Pose, or in sitting meditation. Begin by focusing completely on the physical sensation, form, and weight of your body within the confines of the Yoga mat or cushion. Then gradually extend the focus outward, visualizing your body in relation to the room you are in, then seeing your body in relation to the house or building in which you find yourself. Go slowly with this visualization so that you have a distinct sense of your body in relationship to this larger perspective. Then extend your focus to include the street in which you reside, your neighbors busy cooking or mowing their lawns, then the whole city. Gradually extend this awareness to the state or province in which you live, imagining the expanse of land around you, the many cities and thousands of other people around you—those you know and those you don't know. Then expand this awareness to see the entire country in which you live, and eventually the entire globe, seeing your body as a tiny speck in relationship to this immense distance. But don't stop there. Feel the hundreds of miles of earth underneath you and the infinite space of the sky, the stars, and the galaxies above you. Make your visualization as rich and textured as the life around you: include not only the human two-legged ones, but the winged, finned, and four-legged creatures, the oceans, rivers, and lakes, the trees, plants, insects, and stones. While enjoying the spaciousness of this vision, consider one thing you would wish for yourself. It might be good health, freedom from anxiety or emotional suffering, security, or just a feeling of ease in life. Whatever it is you want for yourself, extend this wish to all beings. Extend a wish that all beings be blessed with physical well-being, peace of mind, safe refuge, and ease. This meditation, similar to the Buddhist practice of loving-kindness, or *metta*, is an extension of the practice of the four *brahmavihara*. Then gradually reverse this centrifugal direction of awareness, moving back from the spaciousness of the globe to your country, city, street, house, and room until you feel the distinct form of your personal body, the sound of your breath, and the boundaries of your skin. Take a moment to consider who you take yourself to be. This practice can wake us up to the reality that we're not cut off from the world.

To believe that engaging in a spiritual practice could change the world might seem grandiose or even messianic. For we form our beliefs and perceptions of the world through our most immediate contact with others: the bank clerk who greets us cheerfully, the driver who lets us in, the friend who listens to our story. All of us can be one of these people. Every day we have choices about who we are becoming. Every interaction contains the possibility of renewing or destroying our faith in the basic goodness of human nature. Maintaining a life practice that tethers us to our core values may not seem such a noble attainment, but in a world raked with violence, divisiveness, and inequity, our life practice, however small, however seemingly insignificant, affords us the possibility of seeing ourselves and others in an utterly new way. One day we wake up and realize this terrible and wonderful world we live in *is* us!

So here we are at the end just the same as at the beginning. The same person—only now awake to a life that lives itself through us every day.

Acknowledgments

A book arises from the body of one's community. I am deeply grateful for all the past and present students of Yoga who have shared this inquiry with me and in doing so deepened my understanding in ways that could not have been accomplished alone. Equally so, the innumerable Yoga centers and studios throughout the world who have supported my work and offered me such generosity of heart in hosting my visits. I am also indebted to the many teachers who have carried on this tradition over the centuries, both known and unknown. In particular, my teacher Judith Lasater offered me a context in which to understand Yoga as a way of life.

The ongoing encouragement and support of my editor, Gideon Weil, offered in so many ways—from cheerleading long-distance phone calls to insightful guidance on the content and structure of the book—emboldened my efforts to continue. I am particularly grateful for the writings and scholarly inspiration of Georg Feuerstein, who has led the way in defining Yoga (with a capital Y!) for a new generation of spiritual seekers. Equally so, my colleague and friend Richard Miller helped in recommending crucial texts in the preparation of the book.

Embarking on this project came at a difficult time in my life, soon after my brother's passing. My dear friend Michael Elsworth helped me through that difficult time, sharing many a dinner or afternoon with me when I was surely poor company. His eloquent readings of the text helped me to hear the words in new ways. My mother, Louise, and my stepfather, Jack, offered rousing praise on yet unwritten pages. Their ineffable belief in me has been a great gift. Friend and fellow horsewoman Chris Jolliffe shared many a long ride with me, and listened to my fears over grooming brushes and hay hauling . . . these open spaces in an overwhelming work schedule kept me sane. And, of course, my four-legged friends themselves, Braga and Tuscany, for teaching me to trust the divine animal that carries us through the world. Is there any better teacher than the vast and wild spirit of Nature?

References

Throughout this book I draw eclectically from a number of central texts from the Yoga tradition. These texts form a rather interesting historical time line from the Vedic Age (4500–2500 B.C.E., "before the common era"), to the Post-Vedic or Upanishadic Age (1500–1000 B.C.E.), through the Pre-Classical Age (1000–100 B.C.E.) and Classical Age (100–500 B.C.E.) to present contemporary studies in nondualistic Advaita Vedanta Yoga. This historical perspective of literature progresses from the poetic and metaphorical works of the Upanishads through the epic and figurative Bhagavad Gita to the finely distilled aphorisms of Patanjali as set forth in the Yoga-Sutra. Although these texts offer different and sometimes variant interpretations of yogic thought, they all contain a similar essential message: that happiness and freedom are our birthright and the only real thing worth having.

The first group of texts, the Upanishads, springs from the Vedas, some of India's oldest scriptures and believed to be knowledge that was revealed at the very dawn of time. The Vedas existed in four collections, each being associated with a family tradition: Rig, Sama, Yajur, and Atharva. These four represent and preserve the hymns and philosophical interpretations of rituals used in Hindu worship to this day. The Upanishads have less to do with ritual and instead focus on the second part of the Vedas: wisdom. The word *upanishad* means "to sit down close with one's teacher," and these texts represent knowledge that was transmitted intimately between teacher and student. This intimacy is reflected in the human flavor of the text, expressed often as conversations between husband and wife or between father and son. Thus most people find the lyricism of the Upanishads far more accessible than the language of the more distilled and esoteric texts such as the Yoga-Sutra, which came later. Traditionally 108 Upanishads are spoken of, though no one knows how many once existed or who wrote them. Ten have been considered "principal Upanishads," on the authority of Shankara, an eighth-century C.E. mystic. The Upanishads concern themselves with a central theme: that the core of every human being is identical with the transcendental core of the universe itself.

The second text to which I refer sporadically is the Bhagavad Gita. Probably composed in the third or fourth century B.C.E., the Bhagavad Gita consists of 700 stanzas. An actual episode of the much larger epic of the Mahabharata, the Gita, or "song of the Lord," is also considered revelatory literature, and in it lies an attempt to integrate many diverse views and traditions. Standing on the battlefield, Prince Arjuna must defend his older brother's claim to the ancient throne of the Kurus but is faced with the untenable position of having to slay an enemy that consists of family and friends. His dialogue with Sri Krishna is a divine dialogue that takes place in the depths of consciousness. Krishna is not some external being or superhuman character but the inner teacher, or *atman*, which lies at the core of human personality. In their epic dialogue Arjuna and Krishna tackle the weighty issues of karma, the law of cause and effect, and of dharma, the complex concept of one's path and duty in life being integrated with a greater sense of justice, goodness, and purpose. Through the use of discriminative awareness, *buddhi*, we forge a path made of self-volition and self-determination rather than chance. Throughout their dialogue, Krishna beckons Arjuna to realize the infinite nature of reality behind the veil of appearances and teaches him that realizing this changeless divinity as the core of his being must be the central purpose of his quest. "I am the Self in the heart of every creature, Arjuna, and the beginning, middle and end of their existence" (10.20).

Any presentation of the subject of Yoga would be incomplete without reference to the Yoga-Sutra by Patanjali. Written later than the Upanishads and the Bhagavad Gita, sometime in the second to third century C.E., the Yoga-Sutra is a distilled codification of Yoga practice composed of 196 aphorisms made all the more terse by their lack of any narrative. It is an extraordinary document that delineates the systematic transformation of consciousness, but it may be the least accessible of the three texts. Although each *sutra*, or "thread," is succinct, the individual Sanskrit words contain complex concepts, like boxes opening into other boxes. Thus you will find few people who have a copy of the Yoga-Sutra by their bedside, for it is rather like reading about the geometry of the mind. Indeed, the Yoga-Sutra makes little sense until one has begun to do the practices of Yoga, and then, through one's direct experience, the meaning of this treatise begins to reveal itself.

Although it would have been simpler to draw on a single translation of the Yoga-Sutra, I found that different translations have particular strengths and weaknesses, and thus I have quoted from five of my most cherished translations:

Kofi Busia, *The Gift, the Prayer, the Offering* (Oxford: Oxford Ashram Publications, 1984)

T. K. V. Desikachar, *Patanjali's Yogasutras: An Introduction* (New Delhi: Affiliated East-West Press, 1987)

Barbara Stoler Miller, *Yoga, Discipline of Freedom: The Yoga Sutra Attributed to Patanjali* (New York: Bantam, 1998)

Alistair Shearer, *Effortless Being: The Yoga Sutras of Patanjali, a New Translation* (London: Unwin, 1989)

Venkatesananda, *Enlightened Living: Patanjali's Vision of Oneness*

The last needs special mention. Sent to me by my colleague Richard Miller over five years ago, this extraordinary translation left me enthralled, for in it lies an attempt to interpret the Yoga-Sutra from a nondualist viewpoint. Indeed, I read the entire translation in one night, so excited was I to have my experience of Yoga confirmed: Yoga *happens* when we get out of our own way. In this translation I found a taxing yet coherent synthesis that tallied with my own conclusions: Yoga is not something that can be attained through self-coercion or through striving. It can be realized only through a tenuous balance of skillful effort and fearless surrender.

The Yoga-Sutra consists of four parts, or *padas*, beginning with a discussion of the meaning of Yoga in the final chapter, followed in chapter 2 by a detailed description of the multiple means and practices that can be used to experience Yoga. In chapter 3 Patanjali outlines some of the powers, or *siddhis*, that may arise as a result of such a practice. Finally, in chapter 4, he brings us full circle, outlining the very highest stages of yogic consciousness. Originally the four parts of this book were meant to mirror this progression, but I found that a greater emphasis on the obstacles and distractions was

more relevant to the contemporary practitioner than a theoretical and esoteric description of states of consciousness.

Last, I have mentioned a number of Advaita (nondualist) Vedanta teachers and texts, namely the turn-of-the-century yogi and adept Sri Ramana
Maharshi and the more contemporary English philosopher and teacher
Douglas Harding. I have also drawn from the Ashtavakra Gita, as translated
by Ramesh S. Balsekar, a text that consists of the dialogue between the sage
Ashtavakra and his disciple, King Janaka. This text exemplifies many nondualistic viewpoints. My leaning in the direction of nondualistic traditions and
teachings comes from recognizing the trap that so many of us fall into on
the spiritual path: exchanging our material striving for a spiritual one. Having experienced the results of such striving in the early years of my Yoga
practice (characterized as it was by self-coercion and covert self-aggression),
I recognize the danger in believing that our happiness lies somewhere else
and that we can gain that happiness only by being someone else. Having
come through to the other side, I can wholeheartedly conclude with my
Vedantic colleagues that acceptance is not born from nonacceptance any
more than peace comes through the practice of violence.

Notes

PART I

CHAPTER 2. MOTIVATION: WHAT BRINGS US TO THIS MOMENT?

1. Georg Feuerstein, *The Yoga Tradition* (Prescott, AZ: Holm Press, 1998), 3.

CHAPTER 3. A LARGER LIFE

1. Samuel Bercholz, ed., *The Spiritual Teachings of Ramana Maharshi* (Boulder, CO: Shambhala, 1972).

2. Brihadaranyaka Upanishad 4.6 and 4.14; Eknath Easwaran, trans., *The Upanishads* (Tomales, CA: Nilgiri Press, 1987), 37, 38.

3. Patanjali makes it clear that none the limbs of the Ashtanga system is likely to bring results unless we are willing to cultivate the virtues of a moral and ethical life. Any corruption in our relationship to self and others is viewed as a sabotage of one's own spiritual quest.

The eight limbs of classical Yoga are:

Yamas and *Niyamas:* The ten ethical precepts that underlie all other Yoga practices.

Asana: Harmonizing and refining the body in order to become an immaculate vehicle for perception. The *asanas* are relatively static postures in which one learns to circulate internal energy. These practices open the channels of the body (through increased flexibility and relaxation) while strengthening the entire somatic system in order to endure greater and greater levels of energetic charge.

Pranayama: Synchronizing or harmonizing the human (microcosmic) movement of breath with the macrocosmic movement of *prana*. *Pranayama* practices develop a constancy in the movement of *prana*, or life force, which is experienced as energetic continuity throughout the body. *Prana* is the life force in all things and is the active force behind all movement, including the movement of the breath. As such, the description of *pranayama* as "breathing exercises" is misleading.

Pratyahara: The drawing of one's attention toward silence rather than toward things.

Dharana: Focusing attention in one place through cultivating inner perceptual awareness.

Dhyana: Sustaining continuity of focus under all conditions.

Samadhi: The return of the mind to original silence.

4. This original concept of the *yamas* and *niyamas* was shared with me by colleague Richard Miller.

5. Alistair Shearer, trans., *Effortless Being: The Yoga Sutras of Patanjali* (London: Unwin, 1989), 49, sutras 1.2–1.4.

6. His Holiness the Dalai Lama, *The Joy of Living and Dying in Peace*, ed. Donald S. Lopez., Jr. (San Francisco: HarperSanFrancisco, 1997), 20.

7. Sutra 2.35: Barbara Stoler Miller, *Yoga, Discipline of Freedom: The Yoga Sutra Attributed to Patanjali* (New York: Bantam, 1998), 54. Sutra 2.37: Kofi Busia, *The Gift, the Prayer, the Offering* (Oxford: Oxford Ashram Publications, 1984). Sutra 2.38: T. K. V. Desikachar, trans., *Patanjali's Yogasutras: An Introduction* (New Delhi, India: Affiliated East-West Press, 1987), 49. Sutra 2.42: Shearer, trans., *Effortless Being*, 83.

CHAPTER 4. YOGA AS A LIFE PRACTICE

1. Eknath Easwaran, trans., *The Upanishads* (Tomales, CA: Nilgiri Press, 1987), 280.

2. Georg Feuerstein, *The Yoga Tradition* (Prescott, AZ: Holm Press, 1998), 9.

3. Eknath Easwaran, trans., *The Bhagavad Gita* (Tomales, CA: Nilgiri Press, 1998), 65, sutra 2.40.

4. Easwaran, trans., *Bhagavad Gita*, 209, sutra 18.37–39.

PART 2

CHAPTER 5. SLOWING DOWN

1. *The Sun*, August 2002.

CHAPTER 6. CLEANING UP OUR ACT: THE FOUR *BRAHMAVIHARA*

1. Ramesh S. Balsekar, *Duet of One: The Ashtavakra Gita Dialogue* (Los Angeles: Advaita Press, 1989), 16.

2. It is difficult to know who said it first. Singer-songwriter Chuck Pyle uses this line in one of his songs.

CHAPTER 7. THE FREEDOM OF DISCIPLINE

1. Gamma C. C. Chang, trans., *The Hundred Thousand Songs of Milarepa* (Boston: Shambhala, 1999).

CHAPTER 8. EMBODIED AWARENESS

1. Eknath Easwaran, trans., *The Upanishads* (Tomales, CA: Nilgiri Press, 1999), 90.

2. Jonathan Miller and David Pelham, *The Human Body* (Santa Monica, CA: Intervisual Books, 2000).

3. Easwaran, trans., *The Upanishads*, 221.

4. Brihadaranyaka Upanishad 4.5; Easwaran, trans., *The Upanishads*, 36.

CHAPTER 10. THE INNER TEACHER

Denise Levertov poem found in *Breathing the Water* (New York: New Directions, 1987).

1. Wolfgange Luthe, M.D., ed., *Autogenic Therapy*, vol. 1 (New York: Grune and Stratton, 1969). Early in Dr. Luthe's research with psychiatric patients he noticed a radical shift in effectiveness when patients made self-suggested changes, rather than those changes being suggested through hypnosis by the therapist.

2. J. Krishnamurti, *Freedom from the Known*, ed. Mary Lutyens (Bombay, India: B. I. Publications, 1969), 10.

CHAPTER 11. EFFORT AND SURRENDER

Meister Eckhart quote is from *Deutsche Predigten und Traktate*, ed. Josef Quint (Munich: Carl Hanser, 1955).

1. Sutra 1.22; interpretation of this sutra by Swami Venkatesananda, *Enlightened Living* (South Africa: Chiltern Yoga Trust, 1975), 9: "Yet, again, it is possible to see a *distinction* between *mild*, *middling*, and *intense* zeal, energy and effort, although Yoga (which is spontaneous realisation of oneness) and effort (which implies duality) are a contradiction in terms."

2. Georg Feuerstein, *The Shambhala Encyclopedia of Yoga* (Boston: Shambhala, 1997), 141. Parentheses are the author's own. Jnana Yoga is defined by Feuerstein as the "Yoga of Wisdom," one of the principal branches of Yoga, the others being *bhakti Yoga* (devotional Yoga) and *karma Yoga* (the Yoga of selfless service). It is virtually identical with the spiritual path of Vedanta, which places a premium on gnosis (spiritual knowledge). Specifically, *jnana Yoga* consists in the constant exercise of discriminating Reality from unreality, the Self from the "non-Self."

3. Feuerstein, *Shambhala Encyclopedia of Yoga*, 241.

4. Samuel Bercholz, ed., *The Spiritual Teachings of Ramana Maharshi* (Boulder, CO: Shambhala, 1972).

5. Judith Lasater, *Living Your Yoga: Finding the Spiritual in Everyday Life* (Berkeley, CA: P. T. Rodmell, 2000), 26–27.

6. Barbara Stoler Miller, trans., *Yoga, Discipline of Freedom: The Yoga Sutra Attributed to Patanjali* (New York: Bantam, 1998), 65.

7. Robert Bly, *The Kabir Book* (Boston: Beacon Press, 1971).

8. Ramana Maharshi, *Be as You Are: The Teachings of Sri Ramana Maharshi*, ed. David Godman (New Delhi, India: Penguin Books, 1985), 53.

CHAPTER 12. TRUSTING THE MYSTERY

Rainer Maria Rilke, *Ahead of All Parting: The Selected Poetry and Prose of Rainer Maria Rilke*, ed. and trans. Stephen Mitchell (New York: Modern Library, 1995), appendix to the *Sonnets to Orpheus* 8, p. 537.

1. Roy J. Mathew, *The True Path: Western Science and the Quest for Yoga* (Cambridge, MA: Perseus, 2001). Recent brain research demonstrates that activities such as prayer, art, and meditation stimulate the nondominant hemispheres of the brain, opening a window into a different state of consciousness.

CHAPTER 13. THE SEASONS OF PRACTICE

1. Thanks to George McFaul for sharing this story with me.

2. See Judith Lasater, *Relax and Renew* (Berkeley, CA: Rodmell Press, 1995), for an excellent reference on the practice of restorative postures.

3. A discussion of Ayurvedic principles is beyond the scope of this book. However, to clarify the discussion on unbalanced practice, it is helpful to understand that in Ayurveda there is a belief that our personal constitution, or *prakruti*, is made up of three *doshas*. A *dosha* is not a material substance, nor does it have form within itself. Rather the *doshas* are dynamic

properties or states that exist in varying proportions in each individual. The three *doshas* are *kapha* (water and earth elements), *pitta* (fire and water elements), and *vata* (space and air elements). Our individual constitution is governed by the balance among the three *doshas*, or *tridosha*. Some people have a strong manifestation of one *dosha*, and we can categorize these individuals as *vata, pitta,* or *kapha* constitutions. Others have two dominant *doshas*—*vata-pitta, pitta-kapha,* or *vata-kapha,* while still others have an equal distribution of all three *doshas*—*vata-pitta-kapha.* And of course, like all things in nature there are subtle permutations of these combinations. While our constitution is fairly set at the time of conception, we can help to balance our health through deliberate consideration of diet, lifestyle, and activities (which includes our Yoga practice) in a way that can attenuate our unique doshic tendencies.

For an excellent source for determining your Ayurvedic constitution, see Robert Svoboda, *Prakruti: Your Ayurvedic Constitution* (Wilmot, WI: Lotus Light Publications, 1988).

PART 3

CHAPTER 15. SLOTH

1. Dean Ornish, *Dr. Dean Ornish's Program for Reversing Heart Disease* (New York: Random House, 1990).

2. Robert Svoboda, *Prakruti: Your Ayurvedic Constitution* (Wilmot, WI: Lotus Light Publications, 1988), 62.

3. Eknath Easwaran, trans., *The Bhagavad Gita* (Berkeley, CA: Nilgiri Press, 1985), 178.

4. Baba Hari Dass, *Silence Speaks: From the Chalkboard of Baba Hari Dass* (Santa Cruz, CA: Sri Rama Foundation, 1977), 131.

CHAPTER 16. ASSUMED IDENTITY

1. Ramesh S. Balsekar, *Duet of One: The Ashtavakra Gita Dialogue* (Los Angeles: Advaita Press, 1989), 16.

2. Balsekar, *Duet of One,* 16.

CHAPTER 17. MEASURING UP

Chapter adapted from "Measuring Up," *Yoga Journal,* March/April 1997.

1. Eknath Easwaran, trans., *The Bhagavad Gita* (Berkeley, CA: Nilgiri Press, 1985), 67.

CHAPTER 18. A BOX OF MONSTERS

1. Douglas E. Harding, *Face to No-Face*, ed. David Lang (Carlsbad, CA: Inner Dimensions Publishing, 2000), 165.

2. Sri Ramana Maharshi, *Be as You Are: The Teachings of Sri Ramana Maharshi*, ed. David Godman (New Delhi, India: Penguin Books, 1985), 13.

3. Baba Hari Dass, *Silence Speaks: From the Chalkboard of Baba Hari Dass* (Santa Cruz, CA: Sri Rama Foundation, 1977), 145.

4. Yoga nidra (sometimes called "psychic sleep") describes both a state of being and a practice for attaining a very high state of consciousness. In the practice of Yoga nidra, one reaches a very deep state of relaxation while at the same time being acutely aware and attentive. In this state one discerns a distinction between the mind, body, and consciousness, with consciousness being the predominant experience.

5. Eknath Easwaran, trans., *The Upanishads* (Berkeley, CA: Nilgiri Press, 1999), 29.

6. Harding, *Face to No-Face*, 124.

7. Rainer Maria Rilke, *"Vielleicht, dass ich durch schwere Berge gehe,"* from *The Book of Hours*, trans. David Whyte, *The Poetry of Self-Compassion*, audio recording (Langley, WA: Many Rivers Company). Many Rivers Company can be reached at P. O. Box 868, Langley, WA 98260, phone (206) 221-1324.

CHAPTER 19. THE RIPTIDE OF STRONG EMOTIONS

1. Venkatesananda, trans., *Enlightened Living: Patanjali's Vision of Oneness* (South Africa: Chiltern Yoga Trust, 1975).

2. His Holiness the Dalai Lama, *The Joy of Living and Dying in Peace* (San Francisco: HarperSanFrancisco, 1997), xviii.

CHAPTER 20. BLIND SPOTS

1. Eknath Easwaran, trans., *The Bhagavad Gita* (Tomales, CA: Nilgiri Press, 1998), 44.

AFTERWORD. LIKE ANY OTHER DAY

1. Eknath Easwaran, trans., *The Bhagavad Gita* (Tomales, CA: Nilgiri Press, 1998), 210.

2. Easwaran, trans., *Bhagavad Gita*, 210.

Permissions and Credits